SPACED-OUT

Baby's Final LSD Trip

By Don Canaan
& Tessa Osborne

Dedication

To my children and grandchildren, the loves of my life. My children include Richard and Kenneth Swerdlow, Tamar and Golan Canaan. My grandchildren are Matthew and Joshua Swerdlow, Rachel, Sarah and Brandon Swerdlow, Alexis Shelton, Aviad and Eden C'naan.

Additional Books by Don Canaan

Israel News Faxx
A hyperlinked index to
news stories 1994-2017

Conceived in Liberty
A time-traveling journey through an
alternative history of the United States

Pretty Little Girl
Don Canaan & Shawn Graves

The Baby Thief
Don Canaan & Shawn Graves

Daddy's Girl
Don Canaan
Prequel to Books 1 & 2

A Giant Shadow
(children)
Don Canaan. Author

Horror in Hocking County
(true crime)

Wayward Pines
An Unauthorized guide

Genealogy for Children
The Bronx Boy Discovers Invisible Ink

Memoir
Gone is the Wind
A child's journey through fantasy and time

Baby sat at his California home's kitchen table staring at Wonder Woman's breasts and lasso; his *Wonder Woman* comic book collection spread before him. As he flicked through its pages, he tried to ignore his mother's sobbing that was coming from her bedroom. If women, like Wonder Woman, were superheroes, then what was his mother? Baby didn't think beating her son on a regular basis made anybody a hero, but he wasn't sure.

A few hours earlier, two men in Army uniforms had knocked on Baby's decrepit front door. His mother immediately ordered Baby to his bedroom. He didn't come out until he heard her run sobbing, into her room, slamming the door behind her. She hadn't come out since.

Alone, ignored, and uncared for, ten-year-old Baby glanced around the decrepit two-bedroom hellhole in which he lived. He hated the way the house made him feel. It was always dirty, and it smelled. But his mother cared more about the bottle, then about her home, and his father was in Europe fighting a war that Baby knew too much about for such a young boy.

Annoyed with his life, his home, and his mother, Baby ran out, slamming the door and grabbing his bike. Halfway down the dirt road connecting his house to town, Baby found his five friends with their bicycles waiting for him. Approaching, he heard his friend Petey, the group's self-proclaimed leader, bragging about the news that he heard earlier on the radio. It wasn't lost on any of the boys that their parents thought them too young to know anything about the war overseas.

"And they said Jews are being *gassed.* They're *actually killing* these people! Children, too!" Petey was saying. "Hey! Frank!" Petey yelled as Baby appeared. Frank was his real name, the one on his birth certificate, and the one he preferred to give his friends. But his family always called him Baby. He wasn't sure why.

"Hey, guys." Baby said.

Everybody in the group waved and made room for Baby in their circle.

"Hey, your dad is over fighting the war on Hitler, right?" Petey asked.

"Yeah, Petey, he's been over there for a few months."

"Have you heard from him? Has he said anything about how they're gassing all those Jewish people? I heard that they're ripping them from their homes and sending them to live in camps."

Had Baby heard from his father? He figured he had, after the way his mother acted this morning. He figured it wasn't good news, but he didn't want to share that with his friends. After all, Baby wasn't even sure his father dying was a bad thing, given the way he sat back and let his mother beat the living shit out of him every day.

"Nah, we haven't heard from him. It's busy over there, you know? Trying to fight Germany and all." Baby answered.

"Sure. Sure. If you hear anything, though, I mean, the Nazis are shipping these people to camps in *cattle trains.*" Petey said.

Baby thought Petey's fascination with the war against the Jews over in Europe was a little strange. But Petey was a rather strange kid. Luckily, the conversation about the war seemed to wane, and the group of boys decided they had better things to do.

They hopped on their bikes and rode toward town, joking about the money they would steal today. Petey wanted to try to buy beer with the cash he was sure he could grab, but Baby liked the thrill of taking the money from purses. Usually, when women were shopping, they would leave their handbags in the shopping carts and turn their backs. The boys swiped the Broman pocketbooks without anybody noticing.

They mostly spent the stolen money on comic books, gum, and junk food, but today Petey said he wanted to try to buy alcohol from a guy who he thought would sell it to them. Baby wasn't sure Pete knew what he was talking about, but he *was* the one who came up with the idea to steal the cash, so usually, Baby shrugged and went along with whatever Pete said.

It was when Baby grabbed a tan and green wallet from a rich woman's purse that a police officer slapped him on the shoulder. "Drop the wallet, son."

Aw, hell, Baby thought. *If mom finds out I've done this, I won't survive the night.* Baby knew his mother was waiting for the day she could kill him. He figured that day was about to arrive soon, what with his father probably being dead and all.

When Baby turned around to face the cop, the officer pulled back as he noticed Baby's bruised face, his ripped shirt and his pants with holes in them. The officer's face softened, and he sighed, "We're going to have to take you downtown, son."

And Baby never went back to his mother's house again.

On Baby's eighteenth birthday, his foster parents gave him birth certificate, a small bag of belongings and a parting wave from them. Child Services had decided, eight years before, that Baby would stop stealing when he entered the foster care system.

The teenager bounced around from house to house, never finding a place that he could call home. He was always lonely. Some of the foster moms were nice, and some weren't. One foster family had a house painted completely in pink; every inch covered in pink – even the kitchen cupboards and the baby grand piano. Baby hated that place.

Sometimes he went to school, and at other times he played hooky He found that some homes didn't care where he was or what he did, as long as he stayed out of trouble so that the foster family could collect money from the state. Baby liked those houses best because he could do whatever he wanted, and nobody cared. Baby continued to have had an ongoing love-hate relationship with his foster moms. On the one hand, he could live whatever life he wanted. And at least the beatings had stopped because he never saw his biological mother. But he was growing up alone, scared, not quite ready to face the cruel world into which he now would enter.

But Baby was just ignored. On some days he felt as if the entire world had forgotten about him. It was an empty, soul-sucking feeling that caused him to blame every woman he met for not loving him the way a mother should love her child. Baby remained a little boy who needed a mother's love and care. He never knew what that felt like but wished he did.

Since he was eighteen, the foster system wasn't obligated anymore to find a home for him. California, pleased to be rid of the nuisance called Baby, received his worldly possessions from his then foster mom, Sandra. She pointed him to the nearest bus stop. Sandra wasn't a bad person; she never knew whether Baby was in the house or not.

While sitting at the bus station hoping to get far from California and any trace of his childhood, Baby opened the envelope containing his birth certificate. He had never seen the actual certificate and only knew his name and birthdate because his mom mentioned it. As he opened the envelope, a letter with an old Army dog tag fell to the ground landing on top of Baby's worn out shoes.

The dog tag was his father's, Corporal Arthur Altman. He hadn't seen it since the day the Army knocked on his door and made his mother cry. He set it to one side, not wanting to relive any part of that day, and instead picked up the letter.

Baby,

I sent this to Child Services in the hopes you would one day receive it. I haven't heard from you since they took you away from me, but I figured the system would know where you were. I'm getting married in a few days, and I don't need your father's old dog tags anymore. I thought you would like to have them.

Your father was a brave man, but he was also bi-sexual and loved little boys. He always hoped you would follow in his footsteps, one day joining the Navy where you could sail the seven seas and put your mind at ease. After being drafted, your father, because we're Jewish, was afraid to go overseas and fight the Nazis. But in his heart, he knew he must protect you and his country.

I guess we've all made mistakes along the way. I know you have, and I'm sure I did too. But I'm happy now, and I'm marrying a real good man next week. As I write this, you would be turning fifteen. Hopefully you're turning into the man your father wanted you to become. I hope, wherever you are, you're happy too.

Take Care,
Mama

Two odd things struck Baby about his mother's letter. One, she signed it "take care," which told Baby that she had little love for the son that, at the time, she hadn't seen in five years. Now she hadn't seen Baby in eight years, and he was sure she had forgotten him altogether. She didn't ask him to find her or say she hoped to see him again someday. The letter was her final goodbye to the chapter in her life in which Baby and his father predominated.

The second thing that Baby pondered over was the statement that the family was Jewish. Baby knew the war was hard for his father to understand, but until he read his mother's letter, he hadn't grasped the desperate need his father had to prove his manliness by helping to fight the Nazis. Of course, his father would want to protect his *people*. His father died a hero. His father died trying to free the men and women from the camps in which they were starved and murdered.

Once the war ended, Americans couldn't believe that Hitler had taken the lives of so many. In the news, there were pictures of dead men thrown into holes after being shot. Here were photos of the "survivors" of these camps; survivors so skinny whose bones protruded from their ribcages, their heads bald, and instead of clothing, they wore uniforms made from potato sacks.

Every day, a tortured Baby re-read his mother's letter, he felt vengeful, desperate to save every Jewish man and woman murdered by the Germans and Poles. In this desperation, Baby discovered hate that he didn't know had existed within himself.

Sitting alone at the bus stop, Baby chose to do something with his life. He wanted to find out more about his heritage, and his father, but he didn't know where to start. The cross-country bus to New York pulled up, and Baby decided to board. *This is a sign,* he thought; *this is the way to find out more.* And off he went.

Baby liked to drink. Everybody who knew him knew he liked to drink. Baby stumbled out of The Tenth Avenue Bar that he frequented and fell over onto the sidewalk.

A man called to him from across the street: "Rough night tonight, Frank man?"

Baby waved his hand in the air, annoyed that this person was speaking to him, and even more annoyed that he didn't have any idea who this person was. He often met people in bars around town and would befriend them for the night. But he was usually so sloshed he couldn't remember who they were.

As he sat down on the sidewalk, he pulled a cigarette from his front pocket, lit it and started to smoke. As he inhaled, his body started to calm down; he stopped feeling so dizzy.

Where the fuck am I? Baby wondered. *And how the fuck did I get here?*

He knew the bartender had kicked him out, but he didn't notice he was at his favorite bar until he came to his senses.

"FRANK! How are ya tonight, Baby Doll?" A woman yelled at him as she approached.

Baby was aware there were many women he had paid for sex over the years, but he couldn't remember their names. Most days he had trouble remembering where he lived. After hopping on the bus to New York five years ago, a time when he was young and full of hope, Baby had stopped in various cities along the route. When he got off the bus in Chicago, mesmerized by the lights, the people and the women, it was easy to communicate and be absorbed into the city's bad side. So instead of continuing the trek to New York, Baby found himself a warehouse job that was posted onto the window of a barber shop.

"Oh, hey," Baby muttered to the woman now standing above him.

"Rough night?" The woman asked.

Baby shook his head, and turned away from her, wanting to be alone. There were some nights where he craved the arms of women, someplace warm where he could cuddle with someone who could take care of him. It wasn't just the availability of sex for him, although that was nice too. It was something people hardly ever did for him.

After the men and women at the Tenth Avenue Bar found out Baby had a decent paying job at the warehouse a few blocks away, they often hit him up for cash, money for drinks or help with their rent. Baby liked feeling needed, so he always said yes. He assumed this woman wanted money from him, but he didn't have the energy tonight to discuss it.

"Want some company tonight, doll?" The woman continued to stand above him.

"Not really, dear." Baby mumbled.

The woman shrugged and walked on looking for the next man she could fuck.

Baby lay down on the sidewalk, wondering how he had gotten here.

***

Baby couldn't remember a time during the last two years where he hadn't been drunk. He would sneak drinks at work, and because he never spoke to anybody, no one ever knew. He hated his life, he hated himself, and even after all these years, he hated his mother.

He called her once, a year back. He dialed information from a pay phone and asked for Samantha Altman. Information said there was no Samantha Altman on record, so he tried Samantha Chapel – her maiden name. There was nobody by that name either. He remembered that she had written she was getting married, but he didn't know her husband's name, so he hung up.

He only called because he still wanted to know more. About the war. About being Jewish. About how his mother could have been OK with her only son ripped from her, and how she slept at night knowing she had crushed the spirit of her child.

By the time he started wondering about where he came from, the soldiers were coming back from the war in Europe, and Hitler's reign of terror had ended. The few Jewish survivors that returned to homes in Poland, Germany, France, and other European countries, were beyond repair. Baby hated that anybody could have ever done that to their innocent lives. He met a man, once, who had survived Auschwitz – Birkenau, its adjacent extermination camp. He recognized him by the tattooed number on his forearm.

"Hi," Baby said, hoping he could ask this man more.

"Hello." The man had answered.

"I couldn't help but notice the tattoo on your arm. I read those were what they put on the men, women and children that Hitler transported to the camps."

"Yes, sir." The man didn't speak much English, but he said, "I left home for a new start in America. I hope never to feel such pain again."

Baby noticed the tear in the man's eye, and he laid his hand over the man's tattoo, "I'm Jewish, too. I wish there were more I could do for you."

The man smiled and patted his hand. He walked away with his head down, and Baby wondered what became of him. It was after he met that man that he started drinking and couldn't stop. He wanted to stop drinking, sometimes, but life seemed so hard. The room he rented above the laundromat was a hole in the wall. He slept on a stained mattress on the floor, and he only had electricity for a few hours a day before it would shut off. He had a decent job, but most of his wages went to drinking and smokes, and what remained was spent on anybody who asked him for it. After all this time, Baby was still a lonely young boy.

At night, when he was hungover and exhausted on his mattress-bed, Baby would dream of a woman. She looked like his mother but was thinner and prettier. She had blond hair and bright blue eyes. She was usually naked, but when she wasn't, she was wearing a Nazi uniform – complete with a red, white and black swastika on an armband. In the dream, she was urging Baby to follow her somewhere. And when he did, he found that she lured him into a gas chamber. After he was all the way inside, the woman started laughing. She ran out of the door before he could stop her, and while still laughing, turned the valve that dropped the Zyklon B gas pellets from shower heads into the chamber. The small room started to fill with gas, and as Baby's lungs began to give out, he would always wake up sweating and scared.

The horror of World War Two had seemed to stun everybody into silence, but Baby, especially, was affected by it. "Frank, man, it's time to go home."

Baby startled awake, realizing he was lying on the trash pile outside the back door of the Tenth Avenue Bar. "Sorry, man. I didn't know I fell asleep." Baby's mouth tasted stale, and he realized he had drunk too much the night before. He hated the way alcohol made him feel the day after he drank too much, but the high was so good when he was drinking that he couldn't stop himself.

"S'ok, bud. You seem to be havin' a rough time." Harry, the bartender of Tenth Avenue, said. Harry was a fat, balding man, with grease stains on his shirt, but he was good to Baby.

"Yeah, I just can't get my shit together."

"Awfully young to have such problems," Harry said.

"I gotta stop drinkin', but I don't know how."

"I can help with that." And with that weird statement, Harry ran back inside the bar.

Baby waited, staring at the door, thinking he would come back out at some point. He dropped his head into his hands, hoping his head would stop hurting. Maybe he could bum a drink off Harry before he had to go into work. Did he even have work today? He couldn't remember what day it was. He made a mental note to ask Harry about that, too.

"Here bud," Harry said as he reappeared outside.

He was holding a small dropper in his hand, a dropper like ones used to dispense nose drops. It reminded Baby of a small turkey baster. There was a small amount of clear liquid inside.

"Whatcha got there? Somethin for a headache?" Baby asked.

"Nah, man. This is better. Don't tell anybody I gave these to you, though. They'd take the bar away from me." Baby frowned up at the fat man, "is it like aspirin?"

"Better than that, my young friend. Lift up your tongue."

Baby did so, learning never to question men who controlled the source of his booze. As he did, the odorless, bitter liquid eased under his tongue as Baby closed his mouth around it.

At first, he didn't feel anything, but after a few minutes, he started to giggle. It was funny that Harry was standing there putting things in his mouth, and even funnier still that Baby's headache had disappeared.

"Consider this round on the house, my young friend. The next round will cost ya."

"Cost me what?"

"Forty-five cents a hit."

"A beer only cost twenty-five cents, Harry. I can't afford this fancy aspirin."

"Not aspirin, my friend. Worth the forty-five cents. Trust me. Just take it. If you want more, when you come into the bar, ask if I have any painkillers and I'll get you hooked up."

"You gonna tell me what this stuff is, Harry?"

"They call it acid, my young friend. And it'll change your life."

For the tenth day in a row, Baby woke up on Judith's couch. He stumbled upon her one day while wandering the streets of New York City, hoping for another chance to score drugs. Since Harry had given it to him seven years before, Baby had upgraded from drinking to drugs; a desperate attempt to fill the empty hole inside his heart that still ached for his mother.

"You're awake," Judith said, not revealing any emotion.

"I guess so." Baby's head, riddled with anxiety, hurt. After a day or two without LSD, he always felt both anxious and nervous, and usually couldn't stop shaking. This, after all, was the feeling that had driven him from Chicago and further east toward New York. He had heard, through men down at the Tenth Avenue Bar that LSD was easy to score in Manhattan. Baby was always looking for new sources for drugs. He couldn't help himself.

He rubbed his eyes as Judith studied him, "You look like shit," she mumbled.

"Thanks." His hands couldn't stop shaking, even when he tried to keep them still. "Are you off to work?" Baby asked. He knew when Judith left, it was easier to scope out the city for a dealer. Judith didn't like drugs in her apartment. Baby was starting to suspect she only offered him a bed on his couch to reform him from his drug-induced stupor.

"I'm not working today, Frank. I don't have anything to get done. Maybe we can spend the day together. I have errands to run; you could come with me." Judith shrugged in an attempt to make the request sound less than what it was. Baby figured Judith could see the pain in his body and knew that he needed the drugs.

"I don't know, Judith. I have stuff to get done."

"Like what, Frank? More drugs? You said you wouldn't bring that into my house when I gave you a place to stay."

"I know, and I haven't." Technically this wasn't a lie. He hadn't taken the drugs in Judith's home, he took them downstairs and came up to her apartment after they were in his system. He had a regular deal from Creed down the street but needed Judith to leave him alone so that he could get over there. He knew he couldn't piss Judith off because hers was the only roof over his head he had. Once he left Chicago, he no longer had a job at the warehouse and had used up his savings. Drugs weren't cheap, and his addiction took all the time and money he possessed.

During a torrential thunderstorm, Judith found Baby sitting on a curb outside her apartment. He was shivering from the cold, and from the lack of a trip he hadn't taken. Judith took pity on him and told him he could crash on her couch. He was almost thirty years old, and Baby hated himself more today than he did when he was eighteen.

"Baby, it's time to get a job and get out there in the world."

"Judith, please, you run want ads in a magazine, and you're hardly bringing in a fortune." Baby knew he was snapping because he was cranky, but he couldn't help himself.

"I bring in enough to put a roof over your disgusting face." Judith looked as if she had tears in her eyes.

Baby's face softened, "I'm sorry. I'm cranky. I need to go downstairs and get something to eat."

"Eat here, Frank. It's easier than begging for food down on the street."

Baby had saved a little cash from dealing grass on the side. Now and then he would use it to buy a burger from Creed's place down the street. "I have some cash. I'll check out what Creed is cookin' this morning."

"Creed." Judith scoffed, and turned away, "You shouldn't associate with him."

"He makes good food. His diner is a nice place to sit."

"He sells drugs, Frank; everybody knows that."

Judith looked like she was going to cry again, but Baby turned away and walked downstairs without changing his clothes or brushing his teeth. He was scum, and he knew it. He knew Judith could kick him out, and he would be on the streets again, but he *had* to be high, or he would lose his mind. His stomach rolled, and he felt like throwing up even though he knew his belly was empty.

"You OK, man?" asked a young guy that passed him on the street.

Baby grunted, and made his way to Creed's Diner, hoping he had something he could give him. Baby's headache was unmanageable.

By the time he made it halfway to the diner, Creed was standing outside smoking a cigarette. Baby used to smoke but stopped feeling anything when he did. He found himself chasing after the high he knew he could get. He wanted to feel the same way he had felt when Harry had first given him LSD, but it was getting harder to feel anything. He had heard Creed mention harder drugs – drugs that Baby would need needles for – but he figured as long as he kept his hands on acid, he would be OK. If he had to, he would smoke some grass until Creed was ready to drop acid under his tongue again.

"Hey, Creed."

"Frank." Creed nodded.

"I'm dyin', man, you have to help me."

"I've got a bit in the back," Creed said. He knew exactly what Baby needed.

"I don't have much money on me."

"Run the grass down to the high school for me, sell it all, and we'll call it even." Baby knew he was lucky because

Creed was a decent dealer. "Bring the cash back, or we'll find you. I know you're staying with Judith around the corner."

Baby didn't know how he knew that but didn't doubt that he had been followed a time or two. He knew people like Creed needed their money and needed it on their terms.

Baby nodded in response and followed Creed to the kitchen.

***

Baby sat at a booth in Creed's diner. To anybody passing by, he looked like he was staring off into space. As the LSD hit Baby's system, he first noticed that his hand wasn't his hand anymore. The veins and lines and tendons jumped out of his skin and whispered to him. The table swayed as Baby's headache finally went away.

As people walked by his table, he didn't see them for what they were anymore. Everyone walking by the table was wearing a Nazi uniform, with a swastika prominent on the armband. That scared Baby, but he also knew he couldn't move. *What if they find out I'm Jewish?* He thought.

Most of the people walking by were women, and they were all dressed in Nazi regalia. Baby was afraid but also aroused. He had always wanted a chance to fight the Nazis for the horror they had inflicted on his people, and now he could have that chance. He sat there, wondering if there was a way to fight them.

"You OK?" asked a woman that tapped Baby on the shoulder.

Baby heard her as if she was somewhere far away. Creed told the woman that Frank was tired, so the woman moved on. Baby hadn't seen the woman, but he knew she was also a Nazi. He knew she was dangerous but again felt himself getting harder. He tried to turn to look after her, but the bright colors flashing in front of his eyes blurred his vision.

He didn't know what the colors were, but when he reached out to touch them, they shifted and moved. He thought that was funny, and he glanced around him to tell someone, anyone, about the beauty; the beauty that he saw everywhere. More women were walking by, and as they passed, he thought about how excited he was. He knew he finally would be able to hurt the Nazi women that deserved what they had coming to them.

***

Baby came to in a place he didn't recognize. He knew he wasn't on Judith's couch. This was another couch, in another small, dark room. It seemed as if his entire life was spent in confusion, wondering where he could end up next. He missed his ten-year-old self, reading *Wonder Woman,* ogling her tits and riding bikes with Petey.

Baby felt better; his headache was gone and his appetite was coming back. He knew he would be OK for another day, but he couldn't let this supply dry up. He still owed Creed a run to the high school, but first had to figure out where he was.

He tried the door and opened it and realized he was in a small room behind the kitchen of Creed's Diner. He had never been in this room before. Glancing around, he realized this tiny space might be Creed's only home.

As Baby walked out he nodded at Creed: "I'll have your money by tonight." Baby knew he already had the drugs in his pocket. He could feel them as he moved. He knew Creed had moved Baby to the back room because Baby was too distracting to his customers. Creed's wasn't a very upscale place, but it still wasn't a place that needed drugs.

Creed nodded in acknowledgment and went back to serving his food.

After Baby stopped by the high school and sold Creed's stash, he made his way back to Judith's house. His pockets bulged with Creed's money, but he was hoping Judith wouldn't notice that bulge. Sometimes she worked late or was at her friends' homes. Then he never had to see her. He enjoyed crashing on her couch but didn't want to be her friend.

"Where've you been?" Judith asked as Baby walked in the door.

"Jesus Christ, Judith. What are you doing?"

"I was just wondering if you were going to come back."

Baby didn't want to say he had nowhere else to go, because he thought it sounded rude. But it was the truth. "I don't mind it here." He finally answered.

"You been doing drugs, Frank? You haven't been back in thirty hours."

Has it been so long? Baby thought. He couldn't understand how he had lost so much time. He knew every time he did drugs; he had to take more and more to feel that sense of beauty and calm that he chased. But he didn't realize he had been out for so long. No wonder Creed had moved him to the back of the diner.

"I was helping out a friend." Baby answered. What else was there to say?

"A friend, huh?" Judith answered. "I don't think you should be staying here anymore, Frank. I can't have this kind of behavior around."

"You picked me up off the street, Judith. How are you surprised?"

"Baby, look, I had a hard childhood. I was raised by a mother who liked drinking more than she liked me, and a father who liked fucking me more than he liked fucking my mother. I don't like myself. But when I see someone that needs help, I'm always reminded of myself as a kid – hopeless and alone and needing someone to save me."

Baby glanced down at the ground, "I don't know what to say." He was confused about why Judith was so up front with him and surprised she was able to be so honest.

"You don't have to say anything. I'm fucked up, you know."

"I'm sorry your dad…you know…" Baby's face flushed, and he couldn't finish the sentence.

"I never hated my dad as much as I hated my mom. She knew what he was doing the whole time, and never stopped him. She had the power to save me, and she never did. She could have taken me away from him, but she got drunk and acted like she didn't hear me crying at night."

"I…uhh… never liked my mother either. She wasn't very nice to me."

"At least she paid attention to you."

Baby wished he could have figured out something comforting to say, but he didn't know if there was anything that could comfort Judith or make his life any different. He was an addict, and he knew it. But if he could play it right with Judith, he could crash with her for the long term. If Judith were as screwed up as he was, Judith would take comfort in having a warm body in her home at night. Maybe Baby could have a home for the first time in his life.

"I'm kinda tired, Jude. I'm going to crash."

Satisfied that Baby wasn't leaving again that night, Judith crawled off to her room and fell asleep.

***

During the next few days, Baby stayed in the apartment. He had enough grass to smoke to get by for a few days, and he didn't care anymore if he was doing it on Judith's couch or getting high on the stairs outside her front door. He knew Judith needed him as much as he needed her house.

He spent his time searching through Judith's work that she left at home on the little dining room table by the window. Judith worked for a magazine, editing and listing want ads. Women or men would write into the magazine, telling who they were, what they enjoyed and what they were looking for in a partner. The magazine would connect them with people who fit their description, and they could exchange letters until they were ready to meet in person.

Baby didn't think it was a very good job, but he couldn't fault Judith for having a job, when he was currently an out of work, homeless, sometimes-drug dealer. He glanced through the ads daily, noticing the new ones that Judith brought home to edit. She was responsible for matching people, and Baby started to find himself interested in the matches. He wished he could see the letters these men and women exchanged.

One woman wrote asking for a man in his mid- to late-thirties or early forties, with a good job, dancing skills and who already had his own home. A man wrote in, asking for a woman who could cook, clean, pay the bills and manage a house. He preferred a woman who didn't want kids because he had money and wanted to travel. Baby wondered if either of those people found love.

A few of the ads were religious specific – a man wanting a good Christian girl, or a woman wanting a Catholic man to go to church. Baby started to wonder if he would put his Jewish ethnicity in if he wrote an ad. Maybe he could request a nice Jewish girl to meet. Baby didn't know enough about being Jewish to understand the lifestyle, but he wouldn't mind meeting someone one day and learning more.

Baby, deep down, was looking for a way to feel better about himself.

When he wasn't reading Judith's want ads, he was doing drugs and hallucinating about the Nazi women that controlled his every thought. When he was sober and lucid, he knew these women didn't exist; women couldn't fight as Nazis in World War Two because they were homemakers and baby makers. They raised future Nazi men who killed innocent people. Baby sometimes, in his darkest thoughts, blamed these mothers for creating the monsters that ended up murdering Jews and other minorities.

He knew it wasn't fair, but his life had become so dark he couldn't stop himself.

At night, when Judith came home from work, he would often talk to her about how he wanted to write his want ad. They would stay up late into the night, on the nights Baby wasn't stoned and pretend they were writing his ad. What would he want? What would he look for? What were the things he couldn't bear to *not* have in a woman?

Judith would cook dinner, usually something cheap and easy like sandwiches or spaghetti or meatloaf. They would sit at the small dining room table by the window talking about all the women in ads that Judith had seen come across her desk; ads that could be a good fit for him. In those moments, Baby would glance up and notice Judith's caramel brown hair falling across her freckled face. When she smiled, she had a dimple in one cheek, and her nose would crinkle. Her eyes were hazel, and even though Baby knew they matched the same color as his own, he grew to like the sparkle in her eyes better. The fire he found behind Judith's eyes was vivid.

He grew to love Judith as his friend. He didn't know if he could ever love her as more than that. But he cared about her. She was funny, and when she laughed hard enough, she would let out a few quick snorts. Baby started to enjoy the nights, laughing with Judith in her apartment, as the sun went down.

After one night of talking about his want ad, Baby decided he might as well go for it. He didn't know why he wanted too, but something – especially when he was high – compelled him to write an ad and see how many women would answer him. With help from Judith, Baby created an ad that he hoped would give him a woman or two to meet; someone to fill the hole in his heart that his mother placed there a long time ago.

His ad read:

Single man seeking young woman to make his life happy! With brown hair and hazel eyes, I am looking for a woman no older than thirty-five to go on an adventure. Don't have a job right now but am looking for something that can fulfill me. I enjoy talking, adventure and reading the news.
Frank

After that, Judith didn't know what else to write and Baby ran out of things to say. He knew there was a possibility that these women wouldn't want anything to do with him, because he had nothing in his life except Judith's couch and drugs. But he hoped some women could see past that. He wasn't a bad person, just confused.

Judith took his ad to work and ran it in the *Life and Styles New York Magazine* the next morning.

***

Dear Frank,
I saw your ad in the Life and Styles, *and I think you sound interesting! I'm up for adventure any time. I think it would be fun to meet one night. It would be nice to meet you and experience these adventures that you want to see more of.*
Yours truly,
Annette

After Baby received his first letter from Judith's magazine. Encouraged, he thought he could meet her, but he was nervous. He had never gone on an actual date before. He had slept with plenty of women, but they didn't need any conversation when he paid them for it.

The one time, when he had too much to drink beforehand, he had actually convinced one of the women to let him choke her, and he had found himself more aroused with that than usual. But, again, he hadn't had to answer to her the next day. He threw money at her and told her it was time to leave.

The thought of meeting a woman named Annette was intriguing and terrifying.

"You *have* to do it," Judith said after she came home and saw Annette's letter sitting open on the dining room table.

"I don't know, Jude."

"Do it! It would be fun for you to see what happens." Judith was encouraging, which was odd to Baby. He didn't understand why she seemed so enthusiastic. Baby had always fallen under the impression that Judith had found him attractive, but maybe he misread those signals.

"I guess I could write her back."

Judith pulled out a piece of yellow legal pad paper and handed Baby a pen. "You have to write it! She'll know a female's handwriting."

Baby's scrawl was almost illegible, but he wrote anyway.

Annette,
I would love to meet you sometime. I am free this Thursday at seven p.m., and we can meet at a little diner down the street from me. Creed's Diner. Let me know if I will see you then.
Yours,
Frank

Judith had told him what to write, and he figured there was nothing else he could say. He didn't know the woman and didn't know if he should talk more about himself or if he should meet her that Thursday and see what else there was to say.

All Annette wrote back was, *I can't wait for our Adventure together,* and Baby assumed that meant they were meeting at Creed's Diner at seven o'clock.

The First Time

Baby was nervous the day he was supposed to meet Annette. He knew he wanted to meet her, and start a new life – a happier life – but he couldn't settle himself. He felt as if he needed something to calm his nerves and his shaking hands. When he reached for the drugs, the acid was there to steady his hand.

He knew he shouldn't, but as the drugs hit his bloodstream, he stopped caring about what happened further to him. He didn't think Annette would be able to tell if he was still high during his meeting with her. He thought he would come down in time to meet her. And he needed to calm himself down.

As soon as the drugs hit his system, Baby felt relaxed and stimulated. He wasn't nervous about meeting Annette anymore, but he was starting to see the Nazi women once again. And this time they were starting to make him angry, like they were taunting him, telling him he wasn't good enough, he wasn't worthy enough. They were telling him *he* deserved to die in Europe, instead of his pedophile father, and that he was worthless.

Judith came home at 6:30 pm and noticed that Baby was still sitting on the couch. He hadn't left yet and was running late for his date with Annette. Baby felt her shake his shoulder, and tell him he should get moving before he missed his date at Creed's Diner. Baby shrugged and stumbled out of the door and down the street. Baby had been to Creed's enough that his body knew where to take him.

His nose, assaulted by the smell of fried food as he entered, approached Creed standing behind the counter. He noticed that, behind Creed, were two Nazi women in their deep black long-sleeved shirts and uniform trousers. He wondered if Creed was able to see them, or if they were just a part of Baby's mind. These days it was so hard for Baby to differentiate reality from fantasy.

"Creed, I have to meet someone." Baby stammered, "I…I…umm…her name is Ann, I think. No, Annette." Baby felt stupid for not remembering the woman he had been so nervous to meet a few hours before. He didn't know why he was acting stupidly, and he hated himself for being so screwed up.

"A lady is sitting at the table by the window, says she's waitin' on Frank. You OK, though, man? You look like you're still trippin.'"

Baby stumbled off in the direction of the woman Creed pointed out to him. He didn't need to acknowledge Creed's question. He could either lie to him and say he wasn't on drugs or tell him the truth and have Creed stop him before he could meet Annette. He knew he wanted to meet this woman and have a chance at a normal life.

"Hi. I'm Baby," Baby said as he extended his hand.

"I thought I was supposed to meet a Frank?"

"Oh, that's what I meant. My mama used to call me Baby, but my real name is Frank."

Annette looked confused, and said, "Are you OK?"

Suddenly, Baby was so angry at everyone for assuming he wasn't OK. He felt like the entire world was waiting for him to mess up. Like everybody was sure there was something wrong with him. Annette swirled in and out of focus, sometimes appearing in front of bright lights, and sometimes disappearing altogether. When she came back into his sight, Baby was sure he saw the Nazi symbol on her arm underneath her jacket. He understood, immediately, that this Annette was one of the Nazi women that haunted him, and that she was trying to hide her true identity.

"I'm fine," Baby said, "I'm not that hungry. Wanna get outta here?"

Annette still looked concerned, but her eyes softened as she took in Baby's appearance. He had made it a point to look nice today – sporting a blue button up shirt, and nice khaki pants he had found at the Goodwill for thirty cents. He had even remembered to comb his hair to the side, the way his mother always liked it. He had made an effort and wanted to be there.

"Are you nervous?" Annette asked.

"I've been nervous all day," Baby answered.

So, with that, she took his hand and led him down the street and around the corner to her apartment.

***

It turned out that Annette lived only two minutes away from Judith, across the street from her apartment. Annette's building was taller than Judith's. Baby felt intimidated by the massive structure but relaxed somewhat when he walked into the soothing blue lobby. Annette's apartment building was run down, but this lobby looked like the residents at least tried to keep it tidy.

"Is this where you live?" Baby asked.

"Sure is," Annette said, "I've been here for four years. Bad neighborhood, but cheap rent."

"Oh."

"Where do you live?" Annette asked.

"I live with my friend down the street. It's her place, not mine. She's letting me crash with her while I find a new place." Baby had rehearsed this very answer with Judith the night before. When panicking, Baby appeared at Judith's bedroom doorway, certain he would come across as a loser with no home. Judith talked him down and coached him into saying something that made him appear a tad better.

"Makes sense," Annette nodded, "Well, this is me," and she opened the door to apartment number nine, on the second floor.

As Baby walked in the door, he caught a flash of Nazi regalia underneath her purse and again reminded himself that he was in the presence of someone hiding their true identity. As Annette's apartment door closed behind him, Baby saw two Nazi soldiers peeking out from her neighbor's front door and knew immediately that this was some trap.

In his drug-addled brain, Baby was thinking of everything the Nazis could want from him. Why they would trick him this way, and how he could get out of the situation. In his achy heart, he realized he missed his mother. She would know what to do; she would be able to get him out of this.

"I haven't had company in a while, sorry the place is such a mess," Annette said.

Baby was once again seeing the swirling colors, except this time they were bright red and orange. The color Baby figured was anger. He was angry, so mad at Annette and at his mother. He didn't want to be at Annette's house anymore, but also didn't know if there was any way he could leave. He felt stuck and didn't like feeling stuck.

Annette rounded the corner, and this time she wasn't even trying to hide her Nazi uniform. The swastika on her arm, was almost as if it was tattooed. He was so angry at her – absolutely furious – that he reached out and laced his fingers around her neck. She was small, so he interlaced his fingers behind the base of her skull, and started squeezing so hard that her face turned red.

As she gasped and cried out, her tiny fingers scratching her face, Baby felt himself grow hard beneath his thirty-cent khaki pants. In a fit of rage, terror and drug-induced stupor, Baby released his hold on Annette's neck and started clawing at her clothes.

"STOP IT! FRANK PLEASE!" Annette pleaded. "PLEASE DON'T HURT ME!" Baby was aware that she had started crying, but he wasn't sure if the sound was coming from her mouth, because all he could see were the swirling red and orange colors.

"PLEASE LEAVE ME ALONE!" Annette continued on, like one long cry.

"Shut the fuck up," Frank said, as he thrust himself on her and in her. Annette cried out again, this time in horror at what was happening to her.

Baby went limp no more than three minutes later. No longer so angry at her for trying to trick him, he opened his eyes prepared to apologize and ask her why she had a swastika on her body. He was willing to reason with her and explain to her how he was Jewish, and he found anybody who appeared as a Nazi repulsing.

As he opened his eyes, all he saw was a young girl. No more than twenty-five years old. Her ripped clothes layered the floor. Her deep brown hair had fallen from a combed bun and was now laying around her shoulders. Her makeup had run down her face as she continued crying, softer now than she had before.

Baby didn't understand what had happened, not intellectually anyway, but he knew he had been wrong. He knew he shouldn't linger and was desperate for a way to leave without seeming rude. He wanted to explain to her that he wasn't all bad and apologize for the terror he saw in her eyes – something he knew he was responsible for – but the drugs were still in his system, and he couldn't decide if the shadows behind Annette were real people watching him. He felt shamed.

So, he pulled up the pants that had fallen around his ankles. He buttoned his Goodwill shirt, turned around and fled.

***

Judith wasn't home when Baby walked in, but that wasn't all that unusual. Sometimes she went back to the office late at night to finish work that she hadn't finished earlier in the day. Or to have dinner with friends she always talked about but never brought back home. This was the one night he wished she had been there for him. He felt like he needed someone to talk to, about what he didn't understand. Even though Baby was a thirty-year-old man, he was still a child.

He laid down on the couch and sobbed until he was sleep.

Judith shook him awake the next morning, pointing to the television set that occupied her living room. It was small, no more than twelve inches, and only worked for the news on channels two, four, and seven, and the vintage films shown on WPIX, Channel 11.

Baby, confused, his stomach in knots, startled himself when the first thought that came into his head was, *I did something bad. I did something so bad. I have to get away from here.* He didn't remember much about the previous night, or about his trip before he met Annette. He remembered dropping acid and remembered meeting Annette at the diner. He even remembered seeing her house. He thought, in the back of his mind, that they maybe had sex, but he couldn't be sure since the LSD made him a little prone to hallucinations.

"FRANK. GET UP." Judith yelled.

The news was blasting from the small television set, letting Baby know that a dead woman had found not too far away from where Baby was currently sitting. In fact, Gabe Pressman informed New Yorkers that the dead woman was in a brick-walled apartment building just across from where he was standing.

"Annette Monachelli was strangled to death in her apartment. Neighbors heard the screams, and when they finally got the door open, they found Annette – naked and alone – laying on her bed. She had been dead for quite some time, by the time they made their way into the house. The neighbors have confirmed the deceased is Annette Monachelli. More information will become available as we receive it from the NYPD."

"Frank. What. Did. You. Do." Judith asked.

The Second Time

After the initial shock had worn off, Baby was certain he hadn't killed Annette. He only recalled having some sexual fantasy play out, but he had never tried to kill her. Or had he?

You did strangle her, Baby. You remember that part. You remember the way her small neck felt between your big hands. You remember the pulse of her artery beneath your fingers. You remember wanting to squeeze harder, Baby. These thoughts occupied Baby's days, yet he was still certain he had never killed Annette. He remembered hearing her quiet sobs as he let himself out of her front door and back into the night.

Since Baby had no record of being *anywhere* except in his old foster homes and had nobody except Judith, there was little evidence that the police could find that would finger Baby as Annette's killer. Instead, they assumed it was a robbery and Baby went on with his life. He knew he might never know what had happened to Annette, and that thought crushed him as he slept. But he also knew there wasn't anything he could do about it.

Then one night Judith said, "I think you should write another letter." They had been sitting on the couch, each reading different sections of the New York Post. The apartment had been silent, except for street noise from the cars outside their living room window.

"What?" Baby asked perplexed. He hadn't thought about answering any more of the want ads since Annette had died. He didn't even know where to begin. He felt cursed like he didn't deserve to be happy with anybody.

"You should answer more letters. You got more responses. Just because it didn't work out with Annette doesn't mean another woman won't turn out OK."

Baby had never told Judith what happened with Annette. He had said that they had talked at her apartment for a few hours, and when he left he said good night and walked out the door. Judith didn't need to know more. Judith didn't need to know that Baby couldn't remember killing Annette or not.

"I don't know," Baby answered, "I don't think it's a good idea."

"It will be fun! C'mon, Frank. You can't be alone forever."

So, on that quiet night, Baby found a letter from Moira. He hadn't answered Moira's letter because Annette seemed more easy-going. Moira wanted to know everything about Baby in writing before she met him. At first Baby thought this seemed ridiculous, but after what happened with Annette he understood.

He answered her as best as he could, telling her he lived with a friend and was between jobs. But his life was so small, so silent, he ran out of things to say after just a few lines. He signed the letter with the intention of meeting Moira at Creed's Diner later in the week – promising himself that he wouldn't leave Creed's place. If he could sit at one of the plastic booths during his date with Moira, he wouldn't get into any sort of trouble.

He thought that it was a good idea to avoid any drugs before he met Moira.

***

Baby had good intentions, but he also knew, deep down in his heart, that he could never meet a woman without having some drug floating through his system. He was anxious, nervous and an addict. He couldn't function without *something* in his system, and LSD seemed to give him what he needed. And what he needed most on that cold winter night was the courage to meet Moira at all.

He needed someone to love him.

He knew he shouldn't take the drugs when Creed looked at him to open his mouth and lift up his tongue, but Baby had a theory that if he swallowed acid *right before* meeting Moira, then maybe he wouldn't hallucinate so badly. Maybe he would still be seeing the swirling colors and everything would be light and wonderful when he saw Moira's face.

Baby could hardly focus when he saw a petite, blonde woman, wander into Creed's Diner. Hunched over, she looked scared. As her eyes darted around, Baby found himself watching her bathed in bright blue lights. He felt calm.

"Hey there. Moira, huh?" He was slurring his words but smiling so big he felt like a cartoon character.

"I'm sorry, are you Frank?" Moira looked surprised, and Baby wasn't sure if it was because he was high or because everything was so damn wonderful.

"I am Frank, he is me, and I am him." Baby didn't know what he was saying, but he found it so funny that he didn't care.

"I don't know if this is a good idea," Moira said and started to turn away.

"Hey there, girl. Just wait a sec." Baby grabbed Moira's arm and found his fingers sinking into her skin. He saw her arm turn to jelly and thought this was funny too. "Don't leave, baby, I'm nervous 'cause you're so pretty."

Moira's face softened. Baby hoped that meant she thought he was acting strangely because he was nervous, and not because he had dropped acid a few moments before. She giggled, turning her painted red lips into a smile and said, "I'm nervous, too." She said like that was the answer. "My apartment is only down the street a piece. We could always go back there and chat for a while instead of eating."

Baby smiled. In the back of his mind, he knew this was a mistake. Something was telling him not to go, to remember Annette. But Baby's head wasn't his own anymore. It belonged to the drugs. So, he silenced his mind and followed Moira away from Creed's.

After walking up to Moira's front door, Baby's good mood turned sour. He didn't know if the drugs were wearing off, or if he was just starting to get tired of the charade. He was now certain that Moira was friends with Annette. He knew, without a doubt, that Moira had helped Annette hurt all the men and women during Hitler's reign of terror. Baby knew that Moira also wanted to hurt him.

His paranoia turned to anger, and he found himself pushing into her apartment. Without giving Moira a chance to scream, he slammed the door behind them and wrapped his hands around Moira's pale neck. She tried to cry out for help, but Baby tightened his grip. He was sure Nazis were waiting behind the closet door, and he had to silence her before they came for him.

As was constant for Baby, finally releasing his pain onto someone else made him crave the touch of a woman. He found himself tearing at the clothes from Moira, then his, before forcing himself into her. He couldn't stop choking her before she went limp, and after he came, he shook Moira so hard she snapped to attention. Her eyes were wide with fear, and she immediately ran from him, locking herself in the bathroom.

Baby, angry with Moira and himself, stalked out of the apartment and went to Creed's.

***

Baby spent the night in Creed's small room off the diner. He didn't want to face Judith. His mint green shirt from the Goodwill was torn, and he knew she would ask questions. He didn't want to lie again and was so exhausted and was starting to get hungry. He just wanted to eat and lie down.

Creed was no friend of Baby's, but he was a man who didn't want anybody to find out he was the supplier for Baby's obvious addiction, so he gave Baby a place to crash. Creed knew Baby was confused about life, even though he suspected Baby was hurting the women he was meeting, Creed also knew it wasn't his problem, just like Baby wasn't his problem.

When Baby woke up the next morning, his mouth tasted sour, and he berated himself for lashing out at Moira. Once the drugs were gone, Baby was sad that he had lost another chance at love. The Nazis disappeared, and once again Baby was alone. He decided he would apologize to Moira. He needed to make things right. He had to know that she was OK. He knew she might never speak to him again, but he convinced himself that she would consider giving him another chance.

As he walked back to her apartment, contemplating his apology every step of the way, he almost ran into Gabe Pressman standing on her building's front step.

"Do you live here, sir?" as Pressman shoved his microphone in Baby's face.

"Uhh, no?" Baby had never been questioned before.

"Did you know the dead girl?"

There's a dead girl? Baby thought. "I…umm…I don't know."

"The police are in her apartment investigating right now. Moira Graham was taken away in a body bag. Did you know Moira?"

"I don't. I'm trying to visit a friend."

"Was your friend Miss. Graham?"

Baby's face flushed red. He didn't know how to lie about this. If he said his friend was, in fact, Moira, but he didn't look upset enough on camera, the police might think it was him and accuse him of killing her. If he said he didn't know Moira, he would have to think of some friend in the building he *did* know, and he didn't know anybody there.

"No, umm…what happened to her?" Deflecting was always a man's best friend when avoiding an answer.

"She was strangled to death. Her neighbor found her early this morning, prone in her bathroom."

"Oh…wow. That's bad. Do they know who did it?" *Be careful, Baby. These questions are too obvious. Who, besides a killer, would ask who killed someone?*

"They think it was a burglary, but since Miss Graham was the only tenant, they can't be sure if anything is missing." "Oh…that's too bad. I guess I'll come back another time…"

"Wait! SIR! What's your name?" Pressman was yelling. But Baby had already turned away and headed for home.

***

Judith assaulted him when he came into the apartment. "Where have you *been?* Have you seen the news?"

"Uhh…I saw it." Baby didn't know what to say. *I didn't kill that woman! I swear it! She ran away from me and locked the bathroom door. I heard the door lock! Dead women don't lock doors!*

"Are you killing these women, Baby?" Judith pressed.

"Uhh." *You know the drugs make you sick in the head,* Baby thought, *you know you very easily could have killed her. You felt her go limp in your hands for a moment. You had to shake her awake. What if that wasn't real? What if she went limp? What if you were her end, Baby?"*

"Frank?"

"No! I left! She was alive! She went to the bathroom and locked the door. I heard her lock the door! She couldn't have been dead."

Judith backed away from Baby, smirking, "You can tell me if you hurt them. I won't be mad."

"I didn't kill her!"

"Whatever you say, Frank."

The Third, Fourth and Fifth Time

Two weeks passed and Judith talked Baby into another ad in her *Life and Styles* magazine. She knew how lonely Baby was, that he wanted someone to care for him. He didn't want to tell her he thought he was cursed, so he went ahead and re-listed his ad in the magazine.

He still didn't have any no job prospects and was still running grass for Creed to earn extra cash. But Judith hadn't asked him to leave. She also didn't ask for any extra money for food and took him down to the Goodwill once a week to buy a new clothing item.

He had a new deep blue shirt for his date with Carol, and he was ready to meet her cold-sober. He felt nervous as he buttoned his shirt and laced up his shoes, but he knew that this time he wouldn't drop acid before seeing her. If he could stay lucid enough to talk to her, he knew she would fall in love with him, for *him*.

When Creed saw Baby walk in, he pushed a beer across the counter towards him. "I think your girl is already here. Small little thing, with her hair in a bun."

Baby hadn't had a drink since the day he dropped acid for the first time with Harry outside of the Tenth Avenue Bar. He didn't know if he should drink it, but he figured it was better than the drugs. It *had* to be.

"I'm nervous, man," Baby said as he downed the beer with two quick gulps, "I'm stone-cold sober."

"I can fix that," and with that, Creed held up another beer for Baby and ushered him to the table where Carol waited.

As they talked, Creed delivered more beer to Baby, until he was so drunk his words were slurring. Baby, touched by Creed's generosity, knew Creed needed his business and needed Baby to run drugs for him. He couldn't lose an employee like Baby to sobriety.

"I don't feel so hot," Baby said to Carol after he had downed his seventh beer.

"OK, do you want to go home?"

"NO! I like you."

Carol was so touched that Baby was so honest she said, "Aw, Frank! Why don't you come back to my place for some coffee? It might settle your stomach."

On the walk back to Carol's townhouse, Baby started to feel dizzy. He felt like he was moving in slow motion, while also feeling as if he was going so fast he was going to fall over. He hadn't had a drink in so long, and he was feeling so good, he wondered why he had ever stopped in the first place.

When they walked into Carol's two-bedroom townhome, Baby stopped remembering anything. His mind went black. His life went black. He didn't think he would ever exist again. He didn't come to, until two hours later as he puked onto Carol's couch. His pants were unzipped, his shirt was undone and he could hear Carol crying in the bedroom.

He didn't say a word. He gathered himself up and left the building.

***

Two days later, Baby was reading the newspaper, and he saw a small article printed on the right-hand side of the front page. It was only a few lines, clearly not worthy of more.

Local woman found dead in a townhome. A neighbor identified her as twenty-eight-year-old Carol Marx. Bruises found around her neck, arms, and legs. Police suspect strangulation due to robbery. Police officers warn of repeated murders within this neighborhood and are asking women to remain in their homes with doors and windows locked. The burglar seems to be targeting young women that live alone.

***

You know what you did, Baby. You know you killed her. How is it that you can't remember anything that happened at Carol's except the very last scene of the night? You know you hurt her; you heard her crying. Just like you killed Annette and Moira. Now you can add Carol to the list. Baby's mind didn't shut off the entire time he was awake. *It isn't long before they find you, Baby. It isn't long before they realize what you've done.*

***

Ever helpful Judith arranged two more dates for Baby, by pretending to be him when she responded to their letters. They seemed like nice enough women, but Baby felt like he was losing his mind. He may, or may not, have killed three women and who's to say he wouldn't kill two more?

His world felt like it was spiraling out of control. He didn't know how to stop it, or where to go next. He knew that he was still the lonely little boy who needed love but felt so scared and paranoid, he didn't know where to turn. This caused him to become angry, and he lashed out at Judith.

She never asked him to leave the house that was hers, and always took his anger in stride. "I know you don't mean that Baby," was all she ever said. Sometimes, she would throw Baby out there, and Frank would wonder how she knew he referred to himself that way. He knew he said things when he was high, and he wished he could always remember what he said.

"I don't think any more dates are a good idea. I'm destined to be alone," Baby said, as Judith tried to convince him Karen and Bette were fine women.

"You don't mean that, Baby. You know you want someone to love you. It's what you're always saying."

"Everybody is dying around me, Judith. Who knows? Maybe you're next."

"Try to keep your wits about you, Frank. You said it yourself; you aren't killing these women."

"I said I didn't *think* I was killing these women. I would swear I was the last one to see any of these ladies alive. Maybe someone is following me."

"Maybe. Or, maybe, someone is seeing these ladies at Creed's place and following them home. That seems more likely in a city like this."

Baby shrugged, hoping the subject of Karen and Bette was dropped.

"Look," Judith said, "I already wrote Karen and Bette, and they are both going to be waiting for you next week. You meet Karen on Tuesday and Bette on Thursday. If you don't like either of them, we can figure out another way for you to find the love of your life." Judith's eyes twinkled, and she smiled so sweetly that a dimple lit up the right side of her cheek.

"Fine. I'll do these last two. Only because I don't want to let them down when they already think I'm coming."

"That's the spirit!" Judith said, and patted Baby on the back.

***

It turns out, Baby only trusted himself when he was high and was desperate for the acid that controlled his life. He knew he couldn't drink before any more of his dates, because he couldn't lose track of himself again. At least with LSD he could be aware of what he was doing, even if colors surrounded it.

Creed, always the eager supplier, never let Baby run low on fresh stock. He was, also, starting to expect Baby to run more of the lesser drugs because Baby was earning quite a few dollars for himself that way. He was almost confident enough to meet Karen without the drugs, but at the last second, he got scared.

He tried to keep himself calm, to remind himself that the colors weren't real. *There are no Nazi women after you, Baby. You have to keep yourself together. Don't leave Creed's; don't go back to Karen's house.*

"Hi, I'm Karen. Karen's eyes were bright green, and her lips were full and red. Her jet-black hair was a stark contrast to her pale skin, and Baby was mesmerized.

"You're beautiful." He said, and even though he was high, he meant it.

Karen giggled like a young child, "Thank you. You're cute, too."

Baby glanced down at his brown shirt. Goodwill was low on shirts his size, and this was the only color that worked for him. He knew the brown shirt made his eyes look dull, but he couldn't change what he was wearing now. He found it funny that he looked like a giant poop, and before he could stop himself he started laughing.

"I wish I knew what was so funny," Karen said, "but at least you're having a good time."

"Hey, let's get out of here," Baby answered. Losing any shred of dignity and inhibition he had before Karen walked in. She was just plain beautiful. Baby knew he had to have her. The drugs made him brave, and his heart made him strong.

"I guess we could go back to my place," Karen said.

And two days later, the news reported her strangled to death.

The same fate befell Bette, and Baby was starting to disbelieve all the innocent thoughts in his head. He hadn't killed Karen, he was sure of it. He didn't even think he had choked her. He thought maybe he had hit her or slapped her, but nobody could die from being slapped.

Even Judith seemed wary. Becoming more silent and withdrawn with every dead female that popped up in Baby's wake, Judith seemed like she was pulling away from Baby. She wasn't home much in the evenings anymore, and Baby found himself missing their talks. But, Baby figured Judith wouldn't want to spend time with a man who murdered five women. Even though he was almost sure he was innocent, he also knew there was no way he could *prove* it. All signs pointed to him losing control.

Realistically, all of Baby's life had just been him losing control. He lost control when he was stealing money from women, he lost control at his foster homes and consistently was transfered to different places. He lost control with drinking and drugs. And now he was losing all his control he had over himself and had finally snapped. He was, at the very least, raping women. At the very worst, he was a rapist and a murderer. Baby knew he had hit rock bottom but didn't know where to go anymore.

Baby Runs

Baby knew there wasn't anything left for him in New York, besides five dead women. And even Judith seemed to be sick of having Baby around. Baby didn't know what he did, but Judith ignored him when she could, and snapped at him when she couldn't. He felt lost.

One night, in February of 1967, Baby and Judith ramped together in the tiny apartment, tried not to look at one another. Baby sat at the small dining room table by the window, wondering if he could bring back some of the happier memories with Judith. *You should try to talk to her,* Baby kept thinking. His mind ran over every possible scenario. He realized he missed his friend and wanted her back.

"Hey, Jude," Baby said.

Judith's head snapped out of the book she had been reading. She startled, almost like she forgot someone else was in the house. Baby hesitated, thinking he shouldn't have said anything at all.

"What?" Judith answered.

"Well, I was just wondering if you wanted to take a drive or a trip or get out of the city for a day. We both seem…I don't know…bored…" Baby let his voice trail off and hoped he didn't sound as pathetic to Judith as he did in his head. Judith's face lit up, "Ya mean it? We should do it!"

Baby realized Judith seemed excited and applauded himself for his brilliant idea. He wasn't sure why the idea of leaving the city intrigued Judith, but he didn't care. As long as she was talking to him again, maybe he wouldn't feel so damn alone. "Cool, wanna drive into Jersey for the day? Just get out of the city?"

"Maybe we should go somewhere better."

Baby couldn't think of anywhere better that was close enough to drive to for the day, "We could go to the beach? See the waves?"

"Let's go somewhere further away!"

"Jude, I don't have any money."

"I have some money saved up, Frank, let's go far away and never look back!"

Baby had never seen Judith so animated. He didn't know if it was the idea of leaving the city, or if she was eager to leave something else behind. *What could she want to run away from, Baby? What could she want to leave behind, except for you murdering those women? She would want to get away if she thought she had been giving a murderer a place to live.*

"You have a job, Judith. We have to come back."

"I'll quit my job! I'll sell my furniture, and we can go."

Baby knew he didn't have any attachments in the Big Apple, but he liked the city. He didn't think he was ready to part with it yet.

"Do you have any time off you can use? Maybe we can take a longer vacation?" Baby tried to reason with her. Judith's face dropped, and she turned back to her book, "I guess we won't go anywhere. You know, Baby, it's probably time you start looking for a different place to live. Talk to Creed. Maybe he knows somewhere you can stay."

"You know, Jude, on second thought, getting away from New York sounds like the perfect idea."

Judith, squealing, raced to Baby and flung her arms around his neck.

They spent the rest of the night planning together. Baby, satisfied that he had Judith back and wasn't so alone, decided he might as well plan a trip somewhere he had always wanted to go. He figured he didn't have that much in New York anyway, besides Creed and Creed's stash. He didn't know if there was a way to travel with drugs, but he was willing to bet he could find some when he got to wherever they were going.

Judith talked about everywhere she had always wanted to go. The countries she had wanted to see. She mentioned a lot of countries in Europe, some of which Baby hadn't heard of before, and she also mentioned Red China. Baby wasn't sure he wanted to go to China but didn't want to argue with Judith and have her ask him to leave again. So, whenever China was mentioned, Baby would shrug.

After a week of throwing out destinations, with no real place in mind, Baby timidly suggested they explore Israel together. Baby knew Tel Aviv was where many Jews had migrated to before Hitler came to power. He remembered hearing about the industrial center of Israel that Mussolini's planes bombed during the war in which his father died. He couldn't be sure, but he thought he remembered his father mentioning a hotel on the beach, a place where his father had always wanted to go.

Baby was desperate to connect with his family. He didn't know if Israel was the place to do it, but it had to be better than watching women die in New York.

Judith seemed desperate to take this trip away from the streets of New York, and she seemed even more adamant that they leave the country. Baby wasn't sure why, since Judith didn't seem to hate America, but he also figured it wasn't his place to ask. If Judith was going to kick him out again, he didn't have anywhere to go, or anybody who could love him.

"Israel?" Judith asked.

"Yeah, my dad used to talk about this hotel on the beach in a city over there. He called it the Jaffa Hotel. He used to say my grandpa wanted him to go there one day." Baby said that his grandfather and his family had even changed their surname from Borenstein to Altman.

The name Altman came about because of their fascination with Theodor Herzl's 1902 Zionist book "Altneuland," (Old New Land).

"I had never thought about Israel. It *is* far enough away." Judith mumbled, more to herself than to Baby.

"So, would it be OK? I don't know how expensive getting to Tel Aviv would be, but we could call JFK and ask."

"I have to find a way to get a passport and get out of New York as soon as possible. Maybe if I call BOAC today, and then sell my furniture in this week's Sunday paper." Judith thought that the airline would be helpful because she had heard that BOAC stood for "Bring Over American Cash."

"Judith? What's going on?" Baby asked.

"Oh, Frank, I forgot you were here," Judith said, embarrassed, "Israel is a great idea. I would love to see Tel Aviv with you. I think a beach escape is what I'm looking for."

Pleased, Baby started helping Judith decide what to sell and what to leave on the curb for the homeless and dumpster divers. He didn't think it would be that hard for him to throw his few clothes in a duffel bag, and he could always buy a few more things from Goodwill before they left.

"Judith, do I need anything to get out of the country? Like a passport or something?"

"Of course you do, Frank. Everybody knows that."

"I don't have a passport. I've never been anywhere except here."

"Well you have your birth certificate, I've seen it in your small bag of stuff. That's all you need to get a passport."

"I can go get one tomorrow!" Baby realized for the first time in his life, he had somewhere to go and with someone.

***

By the time Judith had sold everything in her apartment, and Baby had secured his few belongings to his back in the cheap backpack he got at the Goodwill, it was time for their BOAC flight to leave.

Judith's idea was to fly into Israel and create new, fresh starts as different people. Their passports could get them to Israel, but then they could decide to be whomever they wanted. Judith said she would start going by the name Emily because she didn't want any part of the old life she already had.

Baby didn't understand why their little vacation was turning into an escape from America, but Judith was desperate to play it that way. Baby didn't want to question her any longer, afraid she would change her mind about Baby or Israel, so he kept his mouth shut, and told her he would keep the name Frank because nobody knew him in Israel.

Judith quit her job at the magazine and told the landlord she couldn't afford the rent on the tiny apartment anymore. As they boarded the subway, followed by a bus that took them to JFK, Judith's apartment was already rented to new tenants. Baby thought she was crazy to give up such a prime apartment in midtown Manhattan.

There wasn't enough money to buy two tickets so Baby decided he would stowaway. The thirty-two-year-old equivalent of a ten-year-old Frank pickpocketed a boarding pass with a seat number stapled to it. Both boarded an airport shuttle bus that brought them to the jet-prop on the tarmac. As passengers showed their identification, Baby was able to piggyback his way into the small group by keeping his head down and rolling and spinning his body to avert the flight attendant's examination. "I feel I'm tied to Israel and that's where I belong. It's where my people came from," he said justifying the theft to himself.

The flight to Israel was long and boring. He had never been on an airplane before, and he didn't see what all the hype was. The seats were small, and after take-off, it seemed like a long, loud, car ride, but in a jet-prop.

Plus, the food tasted like rubber. The only thing Baby liked was the cola they brought him in the tiny plastic cup. He didn't get soda much, and the Coca-Cola was sweet and bubbly.

When they landed at Lod Airport in Israel, a frightened Baby watched as Judith navigated her way toward customs, Baby's backpack contained a vial of LSD and a large can of cigarette tobacco. The empty can was going to be the hiding place for his acid and other drugs.

The customs official said Baby would have to pay duty for the tobacco. Annoyed, he told the bureaucrat that he could keep the tobacco if he were permitted to keep the empty canister. The clerk refused but Judith came to the rescue and paid the mechus.

Baby, surprised that Judith was willing to help him, noticed that she seemed to be preoccupied. Baby was relieved that Creed agreed to let Baby deal enough dope to make up the cost of the giant vial of LSD that did make it through customs.

"Todah rabah, the bureaucrat said, and in broken English added, "Welcome to Israel."

Judith found a sherut driver that was willing to take several passengers into Tel Aviv.

She seemed excited by the adventure and held her hand out and introduced herself to the others in the sherut as Emily. "We're getting a fresh start in Tel Aviv," she said.

"A fresh start from what?" asked a man wearing a tembel hat designed to prevent sunstroke.

"We just had to get away from New York, you know?"

The man shrugged, "never been there. Heard it's too crowded and dangerous."

Baby watched as Judith took a small pair of travel scissors out of her backpack. She started cutting the hair from her head, giving herself a choppy, pixie cut. She looked like a maniac, and Baby noticed for the first time that he was afraid of the way she was acting. *If she isn't running from something, Baby, why does she need to cut her hair off?*

"What the hell, Judith?" Baby asked, stunned.

She continued hacking away at her hair, ignoring Baby's question.

"Judith! What are you doing?"

Almost as if in a trance, Judith kept chopping until her long, beautiful, hair rested in her lap, "I had to get rid of it, Baby," she finally answered. Baby realized she sounded sad, like she was apologizing.

"Why?"

"I don't want anybody to recognize me," Judith hesitated, "you wouldn't understand."

The rest of the sherut ride was quiet.

***

After dropping off the other passengers, the two of them, and the driver, continued down Rehov Allenby toward the Mediterranean beachfront and the Jaffa Hotel, Baby found himself getting nervous. To calm himself down, he slipped a few drops of acid under his tongue and closed his eyes against the seat of the Mercedes sherut.

The driver began to point out the different embassies. Baby saw the American Embassy on Rehov HaYarkon and was relieved he could go there if he needed help. He was starting to get nervous that Judith wasn't up to anything good.

As the drugs fueled his system, relaxing his nerves, Baby saw the German Embassy on Daniel Frisch Street, a massive brick building with a Nazi flag hanging outside.

Baby did a double take, hoping what he saw was wrong, hoping it was the illusion of the drugs damaging his eyesight. As he turned back to look at the flag again, it was gone. But embossed on the building's wall, in bright red letters, were the words, *"Juden sind hier nicht willkommen,"* Jews Aren't Welcome Here, followed with a crude drawing of a man with a large protruding nose looking at a swastika.

He closed his eyes for a long time until the words dissolved into his brain. He was hoping it was just the drugs, but now he wasn't so sure. On every corner, Baby's eyes flashed to men and women wearing uniforms. But these uniforms were different than the Nazi ones he always saw on angry-looking soldiers.

"Why is the army here?" Baby asked the driver. He hoped these soldiers were real people, and not just in his mind. "The Israeli soldiers?" The driver asked. "They're here to protect our land from the Arabs."

"The Arabs? I thought the Jewish were afraid of the Nazis?" Baby asked.

The driver laughed at him, "Oh, boychik, the Jewish people, unfortunately, have a lot to be afraid of. Over 700,000 Jewish men, women and children, escaped to Israel before the war that Hitler waged on them. Once here, they received a cold welcome from the British Mandate authorities, Egypt and the Arabs, who demanded their land back. The Jewish have to fight like hell to prove they have a place in this world."

Baby was afraid. "What do these Arab troops look like? Are they here?"

"They usually wear black, with their armbands showing their sign."

Baby didn't understand, these were the men he saw standing on the street corners. He started sweating, "They're here! They're here!"

The driver looked confused, *"Where?"*

Baby went to point out the window of the car, and instead saw a soldier in a tan uniform. He presumed, since he saw no Arab insignia, that this was a protector of Israel, and not someone who wanted to harm him.

Baby stopped trusting himself and decided to keep his mouth shut until they got to the Jaffa Hotel.

The hotel was older and more decrepit than he envisioned. And the walls seemed like they were crumbling. Baby figured it was better than not having anywhere else to go, but made himself comfortable.

Baby and Judith shared a queen-sized bed, and other than a small kitchenette, their room was bare. Six other hotel guests shared the one bathroom located at the end of the hallway.

Baby noticed the red carpet was peeling away from the floor in the corners, and the room had an odor to it that he assumed was because it was so close to the beach. The one thing Baby could appreciate about the small, dimly lit room, was the wide window that opened out onto the Mediterranean beach. It was stunning. He had never seen such crisp blue water before.

And the beach with its white inviting sand was so unlike Brooklyn's drab and dirty Coney Island sand.

Baby was happy, in spite of sharing a bed with Judith who kicked him all night, but he soon settled into a decent routine. He spent his mornings eating breakfast on the beach, and lunch walking along the sand as far as his legs would take him. He found himself losing weight, his legs getting stronger. He didn't need the drugs as much – now that he had found the sunshine – but he still craved acid on the nights when he was in his tiny hotel room.

On some nights, Judith would leave, and Baby was alone in the world again. He never knew where she went, or when she came home. He was always asleep by the time she came creeping back inside. Before the nights in which Judith would disappear, Baby would notice her becoming agitated. It was as if she was hooked on a drug, but one that he never saw her take. Her mood would improve after she was gone for a night or two, and Baby soon suspected she had a boyfriend somewhere.

It was during the times when Judith was mad at the world that Baby craved his drugs. He didn't feel safe walking the streets alone at night, so when he was cramped in the dingy room, he had no choice but to give in to the beckoning voice that acid provided him. He hated himself for it, but after the drugs hit his system, he always felt better.

It was during this peaceful time that Baby noticed a shift in the air in Tel Aviv. More of the Israeli Army was popping up on street corners, and Baby became nervous that he wasn't safe. He felt he wore the word "Jew" in scarlet letters on his chest. He had met a few other Israelis during his stay but had never found a way to connect to them. He wanted to ask them if it was safe there, but never knew how to phrase the question.

After Baby and Judith had been in Tel Aviv for a few weeks, they woke up late one night to what they thought was the sound of firecrackers. Excited, Baby ran to the window, hoping to see some fireworks display. He had never seen fireworks, except on TV. These were a lot louder than he had figured they would be.

Why are these fireworks all orange? Baby thought. *I don't understand why the fireworks are spreading to the buildings.*

The sky turned orange, as more buildings erupted into flames.

"Judith! JUDE! Wake up! Something is happening!"

Judith, shocked into attention, ran to the window well aware that the pops Baby heard weren't fireworks, but was in fact, some sort of missile or artillery. She didn't know how she knew this, but she could tell that the buildings around them wouldn't be falling to the ground if it were a firework show.

"C'mon, Frank, we should go downstairs. See if someone is there that can help us."

"Help us with what?" Baby asked.

"I just don't know whether we're safe here…" Judith caught herself saying before going further. She knew Baby was scared of everything, and also knew his paranoia would spiral out of control if he realized he was right all along; that they *were* unsafe.

Feeling anxious, and hating the way that made him feel, Baby dragged his feet across the room to his small backpack. He stuffed all his clothes inside it, pulling on a T-shirt and pants, and dropping a quick hit of acid under his tongue. He had long ago stopped caring if Judith saw him do this. *Let her judge,* he always thought to himself.

They wasted little time in running out the door, but once they got into the hallway, they were stuck. Crammed into the dark hallway, Baby saw Nazi forces, armed and dangerous, blocking their pathway. The six other people on their floor had their hands up. Fear crossed their faces. Baby couldn't understand why Nazis were shouting at him to keep quiet. He thought the German army disbanded after Hitler lost the war.

"Why are the Nazis here?" Baby whispered into Judith's ear.

Judith frowned back at him and ignored the question. She put her hands up and kept still.

Baby looked from Judith, back to the armed guard, and noticed that his armband didn't have a swastika. Instead, Arab terrorists stood in front of him. Baby rubbed his eyes, confused, and then put his hands in the air.

The Arabs pushed the small group of eight toward the stairwell, with some behind them and a bigger man in front. Baby, terrified, with drugs in his system couldn't help himself when he involuntarily pissed in his pants. The gun next to his back was enough to cause him to lose his mind. *I always knew something like this would happen,* Baby thought, *the world wants us gone. But I didn't do anything! I was born Jewish, but I didn't do anything wrong. That's not true, Baby, you know you think you killed those women back in New York. How else could they have died?*

Baby and the small group of people with him were shunted into the lobby of the hotel. Baby didn't speak Arabic, so all he could understand were angry yells coming from the men holding him hostage. He was finding it harder to focus, realizing the drugs were blurring his vision. The Arabs swirled in and out of focus, and Baby soon realized that if he took his eyes away from them for one second, their uniform would turn back into Nazi regalia, complete with swastika.

Baby felt as if he was underwater, looking at everyone else on dry land. He started to get confused about who had the gun to his face. He wondered if Judith had secretly taken him to Germany, instead of Israel, and these *were* Nazi forces. *Don't be stupid, Baby. That's a stupid thought.* And, because the drugs made him, Baby started laughing at how stupid that thought was.

During the entire event at the Jaffa Hotel, Judith said nothing. In fact, Baby noted that Judith's eyes seemed to glaze over. Like she was sleeping, but awake. If Baby had been sane and sober, he might have asked what was going on with her, but all he could do was stare into her face. He started to wonder if *Judith* caused the raid on his hotel, and that *Judith* was a Nazi, but then he thought that wasn't right and he started laughing again.

The armed guard behind him nudged him with the gun every time he laughed. Baby was aware that the Arabs were getting worked up, because their yelling increased. It sounded like they were putting a spell on Baby, and he thought that maybe these Nazi terrorists were witch people.

Eventually, the Arab troops yelled enough, and someone who worked at the hotel understood that they wanted everyone to sit with their backs against the wall. They guarded the doors and windows so that nobody could get in or out. All Baby could see of the outside world was the bright orange lights every time another shell popped in the sky. Once they sat down, Judith laid her head on Baby's shoulder and fell asleep.

Baby had never before seen somebody die. Once, back in Chicago, when he was new to drugs, he watched a friend of his shoot up heroin in the back of the Tenth Avenue Bar. Baby saw his eyes roll back into his head, and his mouth foaming. He thought the man was dying, but Baby was too young and too scared to do anything about it, so he ran. That was the closest Baby had ever gotten to death.

Baby was surprised that death came so quickly. Sitting in the hotel lobby, during that drawn out night, Baby watched as an Arab guard argued with a hotel staff member. Baby noticed when anger took over the guard's face. He watched his eyes – the only part of his face that wasn't covered – go dark. He saw the brief hesitation the guard had before he pulled the trigger on the gun. And he saw the precise aim the guard had as the bullet pierced the hotel worker's temple.

The women seated next to the worker cried out in shock as the worker quietly fell to Baby's side. It happened so fast. Baby wondered if he even thought of anything in those final moments. Judith had woken up during the argument, and Baby watched as Judith's blank empty eyes lit up the moment the worker died. He didn't know if she enjoyed seeing someone die or she was disgusted by it.

They spent two days locked in the lobby. After the worker was shot, nobody else made a sound. Every now and then someone would drift off to sleep, but nobody wanted to sleep for very long. The buildings outside were burning to the ground. Baby watched as fearful faces fled past the windows and doors. He didn't know why their building was still standing, when it seemed like so many weren't, but he knew better than to try and ask.

They didn't have any food or water, and were starting to feel weak. Baby knew it wasn't the drugs in his system that was causing his mind to come loose at the hinges. He was stone-cold sober now, and scared-shit out of his mind. During the two days that he sat on the floor of the hotel lobby echoes of the winds of war never stopped. Baby stopped jumping when he heard another bang, because he was so used to the sound.

Judith wasn't stone-cold sober. Unless a comment was directed in her direction, she sat there with her eyes open, staring into space. A few times Baby thought she may have said something to him, but he realized she was mumbling to herself. The noise from the explosions outside were loud enough sometimes to drown out the noise inside the lobby. And on these occasions, Baby would try to talk to Judith and to feel reassured that she was there. But in these moments, Judith continued to stare at the wall.

After two days of sitting on the floor, right when Baby was starting to feel weak, the Israeli army burst through the door. Covered in tan, they stormed through the door, angry and shouting. The two armies held guns at each other, daring the other group to drop their weapons first. Baby didn't know what was beyond the doors outside, but he was certain it was as terrifying as was staring down the face of a man holding a gun to your head.

Another explosion rocked Tel Aviv's seaside, flying through the air like a bird, before crashing into the sand surrounding the Jaffa. As the missile hit the earth, Baby cringed as the Israeli Defense Army, the men Baby hoped would keep him safe, open fired on the Arabs taking control of the situation. Baby hoped this was how they took back their land.

As men from both sides fell, Baby shook Judith out of her quiet trance, and half lifted her off the ground. They ran for the door, bursting into the warm June 1967 night. All around them were ruins, the once beautiful White City of Tel Aviv nearly charred to the ground. Baby noticed how the waves from the beach, waves that he liked to wet his feet in, still crashed against the sands. It was almost comforting to him, but then he remembered that he had to run. His people were still under attack, or so he thought, and he had to get somewhere safe.

Remembering the drive in the sherut, the German Embassy crossed his mind. He knew he wouldn't be welcome there, but he hoped he could find the one for the United States. He knew they had to get to the neutral ground.

"Judith we have to go!" Baby shouted. The streets of Tel Aviv were deserted. Only a few of the beach-side hotels were intact. Baby knew the Jaffa was still there, but he didn't know if there was anybody left alive inside.

Judith, ignoring Baby, continued staring at the fire in front of her.

"JUDITH! WE HAVE TO GO!" Baby screamed into her face.

Snapping back to reality, Judith started to run. She seemed to know where she was going, so Baby followed her, stumbling along behind her panicked steps. *Where is there somewhere that isn't on fire?* Baby thought. *Where is somewhere safe? Will everyone here know I'm a Jew? Is there somewhere safe for the thousands of Jewish men, women and children here?*

As Baby and Judith ran, eventually slowing to a walk, the sun started to rise. Baby knew he was hungry, but there weren't any buildings standing. They didn't have any choice but to just keep walking. As they went deeper into the city, they started to stumble upon other people who were creeping away from their hiding spots. Baby didn't hear the whistling sound of missiles anymore. He thought that meant it was OK to finally come out.

"We're looking for the American Embassy? Is that this way?" Baby asked a younger woman who had emerged from a small home.

She didn't speak much English, but nodded and pointed west.

"Frank, I know where I'm going."

Surprised at the sound of Judith's voice, Baby stopped in the street to look at her. "You haven't said anything in days, Judith, I didn't know if you even knew your name anymore."

Judith, with her eyes tearing, glanced at Baby, she had tears in her eyes, "I was sure I was going to die, Baby. I was sure whatever God is up there was punishing me for what I've done."

"I don't understand, Jude, what have you done? You've given me a place to call home, and given me food to eat. You've given me the only family I have."

"That's not what I mean, Frank. You wouldn't understand."

"Then help me understand! Judith, please! You're scaring me! Say something!"

"You wouldn't get it Baby," Judith mumbled, before continuing to walk.

Judith was right, Baby didn't get it. But he wasn't sure he wanted to.

The Way Back Home

It was mid-afternoon by the time Baby and Judith came across anything that resembled an American flag, and another two hours before anybody inside the building was able to help them.

"Sorry about the wait, we've had a busy six days."

"You mean with the bombings by the beach?" Baby asked the young woman helping him and Judith.

"The beach? I mean the war with Egypt and Syria."

"The war?"

"A quick one, lasted the past six days before we signed a ceasefire. Good news is, we've seized the Gaza Strip and the West Bank of the Jordan River. The East side of Jerusalem is ours now! They're saying the Sinai Peninsula is ours now, too, but I don't know if that's just us getting excited."

"I don't understand." Baby said.

"Israel attacked Egypt by air six days ago. But it looks like we've seen a victory now. The Arab army is going back to where they came from."

Baby was surprised he had been stuck in the lobby of the hotel long enough to live out a war. He hadn't ever been in the midst of a war before, and had only heard about the one his father had died in.

"How many people died?" Judith asked.

"Judith, I don't think that matters," Baby whispered.

"I was just wondering." Judith said.

"What can I do for you two," the woman behind the desk asked.

"We need to get home," Baby answered.

"Home?" Judith responded, angrily. "We can't go home! We need somewhere to stay. The Jaffa Hotel we were staying in was seized in the attack, and we don't know if we can go back there."

"Judith! We have to get out of here. If there is a war out, it isn't safe."

"Well, sir, the war is over for right now," the woman behind the desk interjected. Baby glared at her, hoping she wouldn't help Judith. Baby wanted to return to New York where he knew Jewish people were safe. But he didn't know if he could go alone. He needed Judith, because she had the money.

"I don't care," Baby interjected, "I want to go home. I'm Jewish. I want to be where I'm safe."

"Nowhere is safe, Frank," Judith answered. "Everywhere is dangerous. You'll never be safe as long as you're alive. What if tomorrow you walk off the curb and get hit by a car? You spend all your time trying to keep yourself from getting hurt because *you're Jewish*, but you could get hurt because *you're human*. Don't you get that, Frank? It's just as safe for you in Israel as it is in New York, because you can die anywhere in the world."

Baby drew back, hurt by Judith's accusatory tone. He knew he could get hurt anywhere, but when Arab nations were targeting Jewish citizens, he didn't see how that was any better than what Hitler did. And he knew there was *no way* he could step foot in Germany. So how was Israel any different?

"No, Frank, we're staying. At least I'm staying. And I'm not quite sure you can exist without me by your side, my friend. After all, I foot the bill here, right? The only thing you're concerned about is buying drugs. And you can do that here too, I'm sure. So, please, find us a safe space to stay."

"Ma'am, I don't think you understand the severity of the situation. If you aren't going to go back to the United States, then I suggest you head back to the Jaffa. As I said, the war is under a cease fire, and you'll be perfectly safe at the hotel again." The woman worker answered Judith.

"See that, Frank? We wasted this woman's time. We might as well head back to the Jaffa and get some sleep. It's still standing. Do you think they'll have the dead bodies removed yet?" Judith directed her question at the woman working the desk.

What a strange question, Baby thought, *is she hoping they're gone or eager to see if they're still there?*

"I can assure you, the Israeli government is working hard to clean up any damages, including casualties on both sides. If you go back to the hotel and get comfortable in your room, by tomorrow morning the lobby will be clean. I suggest you grab food and get some rest. You've had a long day," the woman answered.

"Well, let's go Frank. It's time to go back home."

Home, Baby thought, *home is back somewhere else. Somewhere near California where I'm riding my bike alongside Petey. Home is back ages ago, before everything hurt and everything was scary and life was so damn hard. How can I walk back to a hotel I don't want to be at, filled with dead bodies, and go back to bed like nothing happened? Is this what people do in the war? Is this what my father did? Watched men die around him, and still had to fall asleep at night because he didn't have any other choice?*

Baby desperately wanted the acid that was left in his backpack, but he also knew that if Judith wanted to stay here forever, he was running low. Should he throw it away, and risk not having a comfort? Should he even follow Judith back to the Jaffa? Why did he all of a sudden feel as if Judith had all the control in his life?

"Let's go, Frank," Judith said, standing up and walking towards the door, "we need to get some sort of food before we faint."

Baby got up and followed Judith out the door, because he had no other choice. Judith was home now.

***

By the time the weary travelers made it back to the Jaffa, the streets were crawling with people again. It seemed as if everybody was celebrating the short war that lasted only six days, and more people were celebrating Israel's seeming victory. Baby talked himself into getting comfortable in this place again, the way he had been last week.

Inside the lobby of the Jaffa, the men and women who had died were covered in sheets. Baby knew the bodies were still under there, but he supposed it helped that they were covered up. He wondered if the other six people sharing his bathroom upstairs were going to be up there. He wondered if he would ever see them again. He wondered if they were under the sheet.

"Mr. Altman! You came back!" The lobby man Baby had become friends with earlier in the trip greeted him.

"Natan! My friend!" Baby embraced him, which was something he was only now comfortable doing. He supposed seeing death stare you in the face made you a different person.

"We thought you would have gone back to the States." Natan responded.

"This is our home now," Judith interrupted.

"Of course, ma'am, I didn't mean anything insidious. I thought you would have moved on."

"The war is over, is it not?" Judith asked.

"That is what they say, my friends," and turning to Baby, Natan said, "But be careful. You never know who is a real friend in this world." Glancing at Judith, and then away, Natan walked through the lobby and to his post at the front desk.

Baby chased after him, hoping Judith wouldn't follow, "Is there another room I can stay in for the time being, Natan?"

"You aren't happy with your room?"

"No, it isn't that, it's just I need some space from Judith for a while. I need to be alone, and clear my head of a few things."

Natan's voice lowered, "is it space from Judith that you need? We have seen her at night, coming back late. She looks dead in her eyes, Frank. Like she's not right. Like there is something missing. One of our staff followed her one night, to see where she went. I don't think….Geverit, " he said to Judith. "May I help you?"

Noticing Judith come up behind him, Baby startled. He wanted to know where Judith was going, but also didn't want to know, because Judith was all the family he had.

"I was wondering if Frank was ready to go up the room."

"We actually found an opening in the room across the hall from you, if one of you are interested? Free of charge for a week. More as a way of apologizing for recent events and to thank you for your continued stay with us." Natan quickly lied.

"I think that's a very generous offer," Baby responded, "how nice to have our own beds for a few nights!" Before Judith could interrupt, Baby snatched the key in Natan's outstretched hand.

"And, I heard Mr. Altman say you two were planning to stay for quite some time. We are always happy to offer you a place to work, sir." Natan continued, refusing to look at Judith.

With the exception of the job in Chicago, Baby had never worked at a real job. Not that being a drug dealer for Creed wasn't a way to bring in money. But this was an actual *job*. And, most importantly, Baby realized he had a friend that wasn't Judith now. Natan seemed to actually want to help him.

"That's kind of you, Natan, but I don't speak Hebrew and don't know any Arabic, so I don't think I would be of much help here. I can't help work at a hotel when I don't speak the language. I'm lucky even you understand me," Baby answered.

"We always need someone to clean. The rooms, the bathrooms, the lobby. They're always a mess. Why don't you start there? Just a few hours a day is all we would need."

Excited, Baby felt like maybe Judith was right. Israel could be a better start for them both. As he walked up the stairs to *his very own room,* he hoped this was a good sign of things to come. He hoped this was the way life was supposed to be. He again thought of the LSD burning a hole in the backpack behind him, and knew he could throw it out. But, he decided, maybe he should keep it, just in case.

Baby's Last Trip

Pleased, Baby settled into his new life. He found that with his regular job at the Jaffa, he was meeting new friends, learning Israeli culture, and even picking up some Hebrew. Around the Jaffa, only a few people spoke Arabic – mainly because of the recent war – so Baby hadn't quite gotten around to picking up many of those words.

Baby enjoyed Natan's company, and a few nights after cleaning the bathrooms, he, Natan and Natan's friend Mikha went to a local bar. It was this night that he learned the importance of always shaking out a towel before drying off after getting out of the shower. Mikha's roommate had died from a scorpion bite that way. The story terrified Baby so much, he didn't know if he would ever even use a towel again. But, Mikha assured him that scorpions were common in the Mediterranean, and if he saw one, he simply had to find a way to kill it.

Baby said goodnight to the two men late that night, before heading back to his small room. In exchange for cleaning services, Baby kept his own room across the hall from Judith's. He got a small salary that helped him buy food, and he was slowly saving some of these lirot to buy clothes and a set of sheets to make his tiny room cozier.

As he walked up the narrow staircase, he saw Judith rounding the corner to come down. *Where is she going so late in the night?* Baby wondered. He hadn't talked to Judith as much, and he wondered if she started pulling away when she saw that she couldn't control Baby so much anymore. He hoped she still loved him, because he would always need Judith, but he didn't know how their relationship would work if she didn't have his life in her hands.

"Jude! You scared me! What are you doing? It's the middle of the night."

"Frank? What are you out so late for?"

"I was with Natan. We were talking."

"I see," Judith answered disapprovingly, "I'm just on my way out for errands." And with that, she pushed past Baby and finished her trek down the stairs. Baby didn't think anybody would run errands in the middle of the night, but he also knew it didn't matter as much what Judith did anymore. Finally, for the first time in his life, Baby was settling into a life he had built all on his own. As he closed the door to the room he called his own, he realized that he was finally home.

***

Against Baby's better judgment, he let Mikha set him up on a date with his sister, Levana. Baby hadn't gone on a date with anybody since he left New York, and he was nervous that Levana wouldn't be the same as him since they were from two different countries. Mikha assured Baby that Levana spoke English, and was also Jewish. Baby found comfort in the fact that he trusted Mikha,

Levana was sweet, young and simple. She wasn't striking like Karen from New York had been, and she wasn't adventurous like Annette. But, still, Baby found himself nervous around her. With great determination, Baby met this girl sober. He had stopped taking LSD, because he found he didn't need it quite as much anymore. He had a purpose every day, between his job at the Jaffa, his new friends, and his own room to take care of. The acid had been sitting on his nightstand, not going anywhere, including into his system. He wasn't yet ready to get rid of it, liking the comfort it provided him in having it next to him at night, like an old friend.

He walked to meet Levana at the same bar he met Mikha and Natan at a few weeks back. He liked this bar, because it offered seating on the patio which overlooked the beach he liked to walk on. He hoped the ocean would act like an old friend, helping him not to be so nervous.

Baby found it hard to talk to Levana, but because she was so interesting, he didn't know what to say. She was a strong woman, but she also hoped to have a husband to care for one day. Baby hadn't thought much about having a wife, but when Levana said she was eager to begin a life with a man, Baby thought maybe he was eager for a life like that too.

Levana asked if Baby had a girlfriend back in New York, and Baby only answered that he had dated a few women. He didn't give mention to the way they had died, nor did he want too. He thought it would be best not to mention his curse.

As he walked Levana home to her small one-bedroom home, he noticed the way her long hair blew in the breeze. He liked her shy smile, and the way she turned away from Baby every time she laughed. He was so proud of himself for lasting through one beautiful, glorious night, without drugs or alcohol, or any illusions that the Nazis were at the door, that when Levana asked him if he wanted to come inside, Baby turned her down. He walked her to her door, kissed her goodnight, and promised her he would call her the following day.

He was so excited that he wandered away without getting her phone number. As he walked home, he realized his error, and wanted to talk to her again. He didn't care that he was already at the Jaffa's front door. He knew if he didn't turn back and get Levana's phone number, he would wonder forever what could have been.

As he walked to Levana's front door, he saw a familiar face walking out of the dark, down the sidewalk towards him. "Judith?" Baby asked.

"Frank? What are you doing here?" Judith looked scared, and nervous.

"A new friend of mine, Levana, lives in that house. I was going to talk to her." Baby glanced down at Judith's hands wrapped in yellow cleaning gloves. Baby didn't understand why Judith would be at a strange building, cleaning, in the middle of the evening.

Judith was silent as she followed Baby's downward gaze.

"Judith?" Baby asked again, his eyes wandering up and down her body, wondering what seemed so *wrong*. Why was Judith wearing those gloves? Why was Judith's shirt torn?

"Baby…Frank…I" Judith's words trailed behind her, as her eyes filled with tears. Baby had never seen Judith at a loss for words.

Baby, wake up. She wasn't here cleaning. You know what she was here for. She was following you, Baby. You need to get to Levana. Waking up out of a staring contest with Judith's face, Baby bolted around her and pushed past her towards Levana's front door.

The door was unlocked, which was weird because Baby had heard her lock it behind him. When he pushed the door open, he saw Levana laying face up on the rug. Her eyes were wide open in terror. There was a mark around her neck, like a cord had been used to strangle the life away from her.

Baby fell to his knees, sure that this time he hadn't killed her himself. He had led the killer right to her. "Levana, I'm so sorry," Baby cried. "I shouldn't have gone on that date with you."

Baby heard a scuffle behind him, and he turned to see Judith lurking in the shadows.

"What have you done?"

Judith didn't answer.

"WHAT HAVE YOU DONE?" Baby shouted.

"Frank, I love you. I've been in love with you since I saw you sitting on that curb outside my apartment. I can't live without you, Baby. I need you. Don't you love me?" Judith shut Levana's front door and crept inside closer to Baby.

"Judith, you need to get away." Baby was angry with Judith for lying to him, but he was mainly angry with himself for not seeing the truth sooner. Judith was gone anytime he came back from a date. Judith was always pushing him to find more women. Judith wanted to help him, but Judith needed help herself.

"Baby, I can't help myself, you know? Sometimes I get so mad at the world, I have to release that anger. That frustration. I'm sorry I used you to find people to release that anger on. I shouldn't have done that. But you have to believe that I love you. I never wanted to hurt you."

Baby backed away, hoping Judith wouldn't come closer to him. He was angry, and for the first time in his life, he was thinking clearly. His mother wasn't standing in front of him, alcohol wasn't blocking his way and there were no drugs making him see the swirling lights around him. It was just Frank. Frank standing there staring stricken at a woman he thought he could have loved, and another woman he thought he needed like a sister. And now, even though one was still very much alive, both were dead to him.

Judith pushed her way closer to Frank and began to run her hands down his body. "C'mon. Don't you love me?" Her hands found his pants and started to unzip the trousers he had so carefully picked out for his first sober date in his entire life. Frank was disgusted that Judith had taken that away from him,

Judith pulled his penis and testicles from behind his zipper and started caressing and sucking them, slowly at first and then with gusto and passion. Frank, disgusted at her sight, wanted to turn away from her, but remained frozen. He didn't know where to go, what to do, or who to turn to. Judith had hurt Mikha's sister. If Natan and Mikha knew it was Judith who killed Levana, he wouldn't be welcome at the Jaffa any longer. Judith had, very deliberately, taken his entire world away from him.

Conflicted, Frank stood there, unsure whether he should run away or take Judith in his arms and let her love him. He knew she wasn't what he wanted, but she was loving him. *She'll show you love. The love you always wanted.*

With tears pouring down his face, Frank picked Judith up by her shoulders to as to face him.

"Judith, I…"

Levana's front door flew open and two armed police officers rushed toward Judith and Frank. Frank quickly pulled his pants up and then just as quickly threw his hands over his head.

The men were screaming at Frank in Hebrew, but Frank didn't know enough of the language to understand anything other than the word *die, enough,* and he was hoping they were talking about Levana and not about him.

Frank didn't want to die. He knew that one day, not long ago, when he was asleep in Creed's small bedroom, he wanted to die. But now, he was starting to get comfortable. And, he didn't want to leave this life. He didn't want Natan, the one who had helped him, to think that he was the one who had killed Levana. He wanted Natan and Mikha to know he was so thankful for everything they had given him.

He wanted to ask Judith more questions. And, maybe, he wanted to call his mother. If only so he could ask her why in the hell she had abandoned him.

The men kept screaming in Hebrew, and all Frank could do was shrug his shoulders, and shout back, *Ani lo mayveen "I don't understand,"* the only Hebrew phrase he knew.

Judith turned towards the four police officers who had filled Levana's front doorway. A neighbor must have heard the noise. A neighbor must have heard Judith kill Levana. Of course, the police were here. It was a silent, beautiful night. A neighbor would have heard if Levana was struggling. Silently, Judith's face twisted into a dark smile. She pulled a small handgun out of her back waistband, shushing Frank as she did so.

The police continued to shout at Judith, and all Frank could understand was the word "*stop.*" Frank knew this wasn't going to end well, but he didn't know if it was going to end badly for him or Judith or for the police officers who were now facing Judith's endless, evil, raging wrath.

Judith's face became contorted into a hideous grin. Her lips spread across her face, and her eyebrows raised, as if she was daring these men to come closer to her. "We knew this would end this way one day," Judith said. Frank wasn't sure she was speaking to him, anymore. Frank wasn't sure Judith had ever been who Judith appeared to be.

Judith continued to smile, as she fired her weapon, missing the police officers and striking Levana's front door. The police officers didn't wait any longer. Feeling threatened and knowing Judith could very easily hit them square in the head the next time she decided to shoot, all four of them open fired on the pair standing before them. Judith fell instantly to the floor, her grotesque smile punctuating her sallow skin.

Frank watched her fall, not knowing if he was pained or relieved. His end came next, and as he watched the police officers aim for his chest, he wondered if his end would hurt as much as his life had.

The End

"Mrs. Altman?" The man on the other end of the telephone said.

"There is no Mrs. Altman here." The woman answered, perturbed that after twenty years she couldn't escape her dead ex-husband.

"I'm sorry, Samantha Altman?" The man tried again.

"This is Samantha, but my last name is Chapel. Samantha Chapel."

"Sorry, Mrs. Chapel…"

"It's Miss Chapel." Samantha Chapel glanced around the house she had lived in for over forty years. First, with her husband, the late Altman everybody referred to her as, and then with her second husband, who had left her and her daughter years ago. Now, she was alone. Her daughter having moved to New York to try her hand at writing or journalism or something too flashy and smart for Samantha Chapel.

"Miss Chapel, then. I'm afraid I have some bad news. Your son, Frank Altman and your daughter Judith died last week."

Samantha Chapel wasn't sure if she heard them right, "Excuse me? Both of my children are dead?"

Even though she hadn't spoken to Baby in years, she knew sometimes she missed him. More than that, she wished the guilt from her mistakes with Baby would stop haunting her at night. She always wondered what she would say to him, if given the chance, but she also knew that it would be too hard to face him again.

Judith, on the other hand, was uncontrollable, and not in the way that Baby had been. Baby was bad like all young boys will be from time to time. But Judith. Judith scared Samantha Chapel. Samantha had been more than happy to hand Judith all the money in her wallet, so Judith would leave her home and travel across the country to find herself in the big city.

Things had been wrong with Judith since the beginning. As a young child, she would find Judith hunched over dead animals saying she just wanted to "play" with them. When Judith was older, children complained that they were afraid to play with her. One child insisted that Judith carved her name in his arm with a knife.

Samantha knew that Judith would have to live out her days far away from her mother, the day Samantha walked by Judith's bedroom and heard her talking to her wall. At first, Samantha thought her daughter was talking to an imaginary friend, and paused to listen to her child's imagination. But then she saw Judith sitting on the floor, rocking back and forth, muttering the words "kill Samantha," over and over again. Samantha had slowly shut Judith's door. She had slept with a gun by her bed every night since then, sure that one day Judith would be standing over her bed, waiting for Samantha.

Judith liked fire, knives and darkness. She talked to herself more often than not, and after the doctors mumbled that Judith was troubled, possibly schizophrenic, Samantha Chapel knew she had to find a way to get Judith away from her for good.

"I don't understand," Samantha tried to clarify, "Judith and Frank were found *together?*" As far as Samantha Chapel knew, the two children of hers had never known the other existed. She had never told Judith that Baby existed in the world, and nobody knew where Frank had ended up to tell him he had a sister. *How did they find each other, Sam?*

"Yes, ma'am. We apologize it took so long to inform you of their passing. We are calling from the American Embassy in Israel. In their belongings was a passport and birth certificate naming who they were. It took us awhile to locate their belongings, and who they belonged too."

"I'm sorry, I don't understand. They were in Israel? Together?"

"Ma'am, Judith and Frank, your children, were shot dead together. I'm sorry to be the one to deliver the news."

Samantha Chapel waited too long before answering, so the man on the other end of the phone thanked her for her time and hung up. She wasn't sure if she was ready to end the call, and knew deep down that she wanted more answers. She didn't know how her children had come to find each other, and wasn't quite sure why they had ended up in Israel dead together.

Samantha had to admit that she wasn't surprised at the reported death of Judith, sure that one day her daughter would cause more trouble than was humanly possible. She was sorry, though, to hear that Baby had gotten mixed up in Judith's pain. Samantha didn't know if Baby was a good person, but she had to believe that at least one of her children amounted to someone decent.

Samantha stared at the phone long after the man had hung up. She hoped it would ring again. Maybe so someone could tell her it was just a joke. She hadn't seen either of her children in years, and had been dying in her house in the middle of nowhere. But, for the first time in her life, Samantha Chapel felt truly alone.

###

I hope you enjoyed reading this book, we would appreciate a review on our Amazon page located at
https://tinyurl.com/Final-LSD-Trip

And please enjoy this opening chapter of
"Pretty Little Girl"
By Don Canaan and Shawn Graves

CHAPTER 1

"Well, aren't you a pretty little thing?" Laura froze. The
sounds of the fair were drowned out by the roar in her ears. It
was already warm and promised to be a hot day, but she was
suddenly chilled and a little girl again. "Daddeee…I'm
scared!"

One of her earliest memories was sitting in one of the
cars on the Ferris wheel as it rocked lazily back and forth. The
wheel had stopped with their car at the very top and all of
Fresno and the surrounding areas spread out from the
fairgrounds, the lights of thousands of homes and businesses
twinkling in the night.

She clung to her father, squealing with equal amounts
of horror and glee each time she peeked out over the edge of
the car to look down on all of the people. It only took a few
seconds before she buried her face against her father's shirt,
the fabric fisted in both small hands.

His arm around her made her feel safe in a way that not
even the belt around her waist and the safety bar locked over
their laps could. She couldn't have been more than three years
old, much too short for the ride. How had her father convinced
the operator to let her on? It wasn't too hard to figure out.

Laura's father was persuasive and used to getting his
way; in his business, in stores, in restaurants, in his home. One
thing he always wanted was whatever would make her happy.
Nothing was too good for his only daughter. He made sure she
had the best clothes, the best toys, and the best education. If
she had pointed her chubby hand at the monstrous ride and said,
"Ride, p'ease, Daddy?" he would have done whatever it took
to get her on. She didn't know if he had taken her to the fair
that first year after her birth, but certainly by the following year
he had begun what would be a yearly tradition.

Although he hadn't lived in Fresno for years before she was born, he had fond memories of the fair from his own childhood. He had been raised there in the days when Fresno was a rural agricultural town. Going to the fair was one of the few luxuries his parents had managed to afford. Taking her back to his home town every year became a ritual that nothing was allowed to disrupt. From the beginning it was a father-daughter only trip.

Laura's mother was neither invited, nor did she seem interested. They always went the first day the fair opened, arriving at the gate before it opened and staying until well after dark. She slept in the back seat as he drove home, but even so, she was always tired and cranky the next morning. When she was old enough for school she was allowed to stay home and rest.

No matter what was happening at work, the opening day of the fair was theirs. It continued every year, even after she entered her teens and her father was the last person she wanted to go to the fair, or anywhere else, with. But he insisted and he always got his way.

The last time she went to the fair with him was nine years earlier, the year she was twenty five. She was engaged to be married in six months and she decided that it was juvenile for a married woman to continue going to the fair with her father. Laura watched the Ferris wheel, remembering. She remembered the exhilaration of rising in the air, the way her stomach did flip-flops as they descended. Most of all, she remembered being three years old.

She remembered thinking her father was the biggest, strongest, bravest man in the world. She remembered that feeling of assurance that nothing could hurt her as long as he was holding her. She looked over at him now. It was the first day of the fair and she was there once again with her father.

He didn't look big, or strong, or particularly brave. Today he just seemed…lost. His hair was white; he didn't stand as straight as she remembered from her childhood. He certainly didn't exude the confidence and authority that had always convinced everyone from powerful CEOs to Ferris wheel operators to accede to his wishes. "Daddy, do you remember taking me on the Ferris wheel?" He smiled at her. "I think there's time for nine holes before that meeting." "Dad, we aren't at the golf course. We're at the fair. Remember? The Fresno Fair? You and I used to come every year." "I just need to pick up my clubs."

He ambled away and Laura followed a few feet behind, watching him stop to bend down and pick up an imaginary tee. The exhaustion of the last two years suddenly settled over her, along with the familiar resentment of having put her life on hold. The life that had fallen apart.

As they neared the exhibit halls, she caught up to him. "Dad, do you want something to eat?" "We have a foursome and it's too beautiful a day to waste indoors." "You don't even know who I am, do you," she sighed. He patted her hand where it rested on his arm. "Well, aren't you a pretty little thing?"

Laura released his arm as he knelt to put the imaginary tee in the dirt. Reaching into her purse, she ripped a piece of paper from her notebook and located a pen. She quickly wrote on the paper and when he stood up, she folded the paper and tucked it into the breast pocket of his shirt.

"The boys want to meet in the bar for drinks before we start," he told her. "The clubhouse is right over there," she replied, pointing to the Home Arts Building just across the grass. He smiled and headed in that direction. She watched him, knowing that within a few steps he had already forgotten where he was going. The tide of people broke around her as she stood, feeling her heart pound in her chest. He followed the crowd of people moving toward the building. He stepped through the large open doors and into the shade. The crowd closed around him and then her father disappeared from her sight. Still she stood there, her eyes watching the doorway.

For five minutes she waited, and then she pulled the strap of her purse onto her shoulder and began walking away from the building. She walked to a different gate from the one they had entered less than an hour earlier. Refusing a stamp on her wrist that would allow her to reenter the fairgrounds later, she slipped through the exit. She walked to the parking lot where she had parked her car.

Sliding behind the wheel, she started the car and turned the air conditioning on. Taking a deep breath, she closed her eyes and rested her forehead against the steering wheel for several moments. Finally, she backed out of the parking space, and pulled out onto Chance Avenue. She made her way slowly through the busy streets until she found the entrance to Highway 41. Merging into the southbound lanes, Laura drove away from Fresno. Away from her memories. "Well, aren't you a pretty little thing?"

The Authors
Don Canaan

Life is cyclical. Everything, fashion, music, economics --
eventually return. And so did Don Canaan -- from a Bronx
tenement to marriage, children, success in television news film,
immigration to Israel, re-marriage, two more children and a
return to the U.S.A. and a new facet of journalism--print.

Canaan's career and news background covers four
decades of history -- from 1960 until his departure from United
Press International to become a Quality Editor for LexisNexis.

From 1961-1974, Canaan edited news film and
documentaries for NBC News in New York, and in 1974
immigrated to Israel as part of an American group planning to
settle the new Sinai city of Yamit.

When he returned to the U.S., film in TV news had
become an anachronism. During three years overseas, 17 years
of TV film journalism experience disappeared.

The Ohio State University's School of Journalism in
Columbus, Ohio, came to the rescue with an offer to earn a
Master's Degree in Journalism, while serving as an assistant in
its TV news workshop.

An opportunity materialized at the American Israelite
in Cincinnati where he served as reporter, editor and
photographer.

Canaan's four-part series, "Jews in Ohio's Prisons:
Does Anybody Care?" received a first place award for best
weekly journalism in Ohio from the State of Ohio Bar
Association.

Currently, Canaan compiles and edits Israel News Faxx,
a newsletter sent to clients around the world. Past issues are
archived in various databases and at

Tessa Osborne

Tessa Osborne is a trained editor and creative writer. After studying for her Bachelor's Degree in English Literature, Tessa spent the next year working with local businesses in Reno, Nevada to provide interesting blog and website content.

Tessa currently writes weekly blog posts and essays for The Yoga Pearl, as well as her own website The Monkey Mind Mom. She is currently working toward her Master's Degree in English, and hopes to continue sharing her love of words with the world. Tessa lives in Reno, Nevada with two cats, two dogs, two kids and one husband.